LIFESTYLE RESET

Post Covid

KANCHAN VERMA

BlueRose ONE.com
Stories Matter
NewDelhi • London

BLUEROSE PUBLISHERS
India | U.K.

BlueRose ONE.com
Stories Matter
NewDelhi • London

For permissions requests or inquiries regarding this publication, please contact:

BLUEROSE PUBLISHERS
www.BlueRoseONE.com
info@bluerosepublishers.com
+91 8882 898 898
+4407342408967

ISBN: 978-93-5628-053-3

Cover design: Yash Singhal
Typesetting: Namrata Saini

First Edition: June 2025

Acknowledgment

As I write these final words, my heart is filled with gratitude—for the wisdom of the past, for the healing of the present, and for the transformation yet to come. This book is more than just a guide; it is a promise—a promise that change is possible, that healing is within reach, and that you are stronger than the struggles you face. To those who have supported me along the way—family, friends, mentors, and wellness experts—your encouragement and wisdom have been instrumental in shaping this work. I know the weight of exhaustion, the frustration of trying everything and still feeling lost. I know what it means to seek answers in a world full of noise. But I also know the power of stillness, the magic of breath, the quiet strength that comes from listening to your body rather than fighting against it. And that is why this book exists—to remind you that you are not alone on this journey. Each time you step onto your mat, each time you take a mindful breath, each time you nourish your body with the right foods, you are reclaiming your health, one choice at a time. Healing is not a race. It is a gentle unfolding, a return to the wholeness that has always been within you. So, as you move forward, be patient with yourself. Celebrate the small victories. If you stumble, do not turn back—just take the next step. Change is not about perfection; it is about consistency, about showing up for yourself even on the hardest days. To my readers—this book belongs to you now. May it hold your hand in moments of doubt, may it remind you of your own strength, and may it be the beginning of a new chapter—one filled with light, balance, and the deep knowing that you are capable of healing, of thriving, of living fully.

With all my heart,
[Kanchan Verma]

Prologue

A Journey from Chaos to Calm: My Path to Becoming a Yoga Sadika

Life before yoga was a whirlwind—busy, unpredictable, and overwhelming. I had earned an MBA in HR and was working as the Head of Talent Acquisition in the corporate sector. When I married an Army officer, a whole new chapter began. Being married to a man in uniform brings immense pride, but it also comes with a unique set of challenges. One of the toughest parts was constantly relocating—packing up our lives and moving to a new city, a new environment, time and time again.

Two years into the corporate grind, I made a bold decision. I quit. It was a leap into the unknown, but I was searching for something deeper—something that my corporate job just couldn't offer. However, leaving my job didn't mean the chaos disappeared. I was now juggling more—moving from city to city, trying to settle into each new place while dealing with the emotional toll it took on me.

Three years later, I experienced one of life's greatest joys: becoming a mother. But motherhood, like everything else, brought its own set of challenges. Weight gain, PCOS, thyroid issues, and eventually postpartum depression started to weigh me down. The sleepless nights and constant fatigue were exhausting, and I found myself in a place I never thought I'd be—struggling with my health, my confidence, and my mental well-being.

I wasn't the vibrant, active woman I used to be. Instead, I was tired all the time, plagued by mood swings, and wrestling with the demands of motherhood and my own body. The confidence I once had faded, and the stress of balancing life, work, and family took a toll on both my body and mind.

In the darkest moments, I clung to the only solution I knew—fitness. I went back to the gym, tried Zumba again, and threw myself into CrossFit training. But despite all my efforts, I felt like I was only addressing one part of the problem. My mind was still restless, and the surrounding chaos didn't subside.

It was then that yoga came into my life, as my destiny. My mother suggested it, and though I was skeptical at first, something inside me said, Let's try! This choice marked the beginning of a journey that would completely change me, both mentally and physically.

Those first few days on the mat were awkward. My body was stiff, and I struggled with the poses, much like I was struggling in life. But as I persisted, something began to shift. The constant ticking in my mind—the relentless, anxious thoughts—started to fade. Slowly but surely, yoga became my sanctuary, a place where I could find peace amidst the chaos.

It wasn't just the physical practice that helped; it was the stillness, the mindfulness, the connection between breath and movement. Yoga became my anchor, and through its discipline, I started to rediscover myself. My circumstances hadn't changed—I was still moving from city to city, raising a child, and dealing with the demands of life. But the way I handled those challenges had shifted. Yoga gave me the strength and clarity I needed to face life head-on.

As I deepened my practice, I realised that yoga wasn't just a temporary escape from stress—it was a lifestyle, a way of aligning my body, mind, and soul. I started reading more about yoga, studying its different forms, and learning about its healing power. But books and articles weren't enough to quench my thirst for knowledge. I wanted to go deeper, to understand how yoga heals.

That's when I enrolled in a Yoga Therapy course with the AYUSH Ministry. The training was eye-opening, teaching me how yoga could prevent lifestyle diseases rather than just treat them. I learned that true health isn't about quick fixes or temporary relief; it's about building a sustainable ecosystem for both the body and the mind.

Today, as a certified Yoga Therapist, I've dedicated my life to sharing this knowledge with others. Yoga has not only healed my body but also my spirit. It has shown me that we have the power to reset our lives, no matter how chaotic things may seem. Through mindful movement and meditation, I've reclaimed my sense of self, found peace amidst the storms, and rediscovered the vibrant, active woman I once was.

If you find yourself lost in the whirlwind of life, take a moment to breathe. Start small—maybe with just a few minutes on the mat. You'll be amazed at how something so simple can change everything. Yoga isn't just a practice; it's a way of life. And for me, it has been the key to unlocking a healthier, more balanced, and empowered version of myself. Through this book, you will discover the true essence of yoga—not just as a practice but as a powerful tool for healing. You will uncover the rich history of yoga, understand how it influences the 13 organ systems and the pineal gland, and most importantly, learn how to create a yoga routine that helps you prevent and reverse lifestyle diseases naturally.

At the heart of this transformation lies the 5-Day Lifestyle Reset Program, a holistic approach designed to reset your gut, rejuvenate your body, and refresh your mind. This journey will take you through:

🌱 Gut Reset – Cleansing and nourishing your digestive system for optimal health.
💪 Body Reset – Detoxifying and strengthening your physical being through mindful movement.
🧘 Mind Reset – Cultivating inner peace and mental clarity to break free from stress.
🥗 Viprit Ahaar – Understanding food beyond nutrition, embracing balance and compatibility.
✨ Dry Brushing for Immunity – Awakening your lymphatic system and boosting natural defences.

Every chapter, every practice, and every insight shared in this book is a step towards your healing—a way to reconnect with yourself and live a life of vitality, joy, and true well-being.

Are you ready to reset your life and reclaim your health? Your transformation starts now. 💫

Title	Description
Introduction to Yoga: A Path to Wellness	Discover the fundamentals of yoga and how it enhances physical, mental, and spiritual well-being.

Transform your Life with Yoga: Key Benefits Unveiled	Explore how practicing yoga can transform your health, reduce stress, and improve daily life.
Yoga & Your Body: How It Supports 11 Vital Organ Systems	Learn how yoga influences and benefits all 11 organ systems, promoting overall wellness.
The Pineal Gland Mystery: Unlocking Your Inner Light	Discover the role of the pineal gland in spiritual awakening and inner balance.
Building Your Yoga Routine: A Step-by-Step Guide	Learn how to establish a consistent yoga practice that fits your lifestyle and goals.
The 5-Day Lifestyle Reset: Renew, Recharge, Rebalance	Refresh your body and mind with a structured 5-day yoga plan for renewal and growth.
Let's Get Started: Your Yoga Journey Begins	Take the first step towards a healthier, balanced life with given asanas, pranayam and meditation.

Contents

Chapter 1
Introduction to Yoga: A Path to Wellness

During my journey of being a Yoga Therapist, I read this beautiful shloka which defines a healthy person written in Sanskrit that too Approx. 5000 years ago.

(Sushrut Samhita, Sutrasthan, Ch. 15, Shloka 10) According to ancient Ayurvedist Maharishi Sushruta

समाग्निश्च समधातुमलक्रियः / प्रसन्न आत्मेन्द्रियेमनाः स्वस्थ इत्यभिधीयते

This means when an individual/person who is in a state of equilibrium of body's digestive fire, when dhatus are in equilibrium i.e plasma, blood, muscle, fat, bone, bone marrow and reproductive fluid, Then there is timely excretion of the waste from the body.

Not just this, now shloka explains that its also significant to have blissful soul, Content senses and a peaceful mind. This is the complete definition of a healthy person given in 1200 B.C

The ancient wisdom that defined health over 3,000- 5000 years ago is nothing short of remarkable, both in its depth and scientific insight. Imagine, in 1200 B.C., our ancestors already understood that true health transcends not merely through physical well-being. They recognised that the body's internal balance—what they referred to as the equilibrium of the digestive fire and the dhatus (the essential tissues like plasma, blood, muscle, and more)—was crucial for maintaining vitality. This understanding is incredibly advanced, as it aligns closely with modern concepts of homeostasis and metabolic health, which are central to contemporary medicine.

But they didn't stop there. The ancient sages knew that health wasn't just about the physical body. They emphasised the importance of timely excretion, which today we understand as the body's detoxification processes—a key component of preventing illness and maintaining health. This holistic view, integrating physical processes with the need for mental and spiritual well-being, is where their knowledge truly shines.

The inclusion of a "blissful soul, content senses, and peaceful mind" in their definition of health reveals an understanding that well-being is multifaceted. It's not just the absence of disease but a state of harmony within the body, mind, and spirit. This holistic approach is something modern science is only now beginning to fully appreciate, as we understand the profound impact that mental and emotional health has on physical health.

This ancient knowledge was not only incredible for its time but also remarkably scientific, as it recognised the intricate connections between different aspects of human health. It's a testament to the profound wisdom of our ancestors, whose teachings continue to inspire and guide us in our pursuit of true well-being even today.

While

The definition by WHO constitution states: "Health is a state of complete physical, mental and social well-being and not merely the absence of disease or infirmity." Which is still incomplete in many sense till now. That too in the year 2025.

What's truly astonishing is how these ancient teachings anticipated the interconnectedness of body, mind, and spirit—a concept that modern science is increasingly validating. But not able to give you ways to do it. And it is significant for you to change your lifestyle to captured this holistic view of health before you start dealing with lifestyle diseases.

Today, you understand that the state of your mental health can directly impact your physical health, and vice versa. Stress, anxiety, and emotional turmoil can manifest in physical symptoms, just as physical ailments can lead to mental distress. The ancient wisdom consider the emphasis on the digestive fire, or Agni, as it was known in ancient texts. This concept parallels what you now know about metabolism and gut health.

Modern research has revealed that the gut is often referred to as the "second brain," with its complex system of nerves and connections that communicate with the brain, affecting everything from mood to immunity. The ancient sages recognised the importance of a balanced digestive fire in maintaining overall health, understanding that when digestion is optimal, the body's tissues are nourished, waste is efficiently removed, and energy flows freely.

Furthermore, the ancient texts didn't just focus on the physical but also placed immense value on the state of the soul, the senses, and the mind. A blissful soul, they taught, is essential for true health. Today, you might equate this to emotional well-being or a sense of purpose, both of which are now recognised as critical components of health. Similarly, content senses—what you might now call sensory balance or harmony—highlight the need for a lifestyle that doesn't overstimulate or dull your senses but instead nurtures them in a balanced way.

The peaceful mind, too, is a concept that resonates deeply with modern psychological and neurological science. You now know that chronic stress and a disturbed mind can lead to a host of physical ailments, including heart disease, diabetes, and autoimmune disorders. The ancient understanding that a peaceful mind is integral to health shows a profound grasp of what it takes to maintain overall well-being.

The ancient definition of health was a holistic, interconnected vision that remains highly relevant today. It wasn't just about the absence of disease; it was about achieving a state of complete harmony within oneself. This wisdom reflects an advanced understanding of the human condition, one that modern science is only beginning to fully appreciate. It serves as a powerful reminder that the path to true health lies in balancing all aspects of your being—physical, mental, and spiritual—just as your ancestors so wisely understood. Because, its important for you to have a life which is Balanced, fulfilling and wholesome.

The fundamental query emerges: how? When emotions propel you from the moment you rise in the morning until you retire at night, each action becomes a reflection of your prevailing emotional state. Effective communication typically signals a positive emotional state, while the inverse suggests a presence of negative emotions such as anger, jealousy, disgust, guilt, or nervousness.

In essence, your emotions serve as the linchpin for your actions and decisions. The question then becomes: how can you navigate and influence them? It requires identifying the actions and decisions driven by your current emotional state, fostering self-awareness in those moments.

Self-awareness through yoga is cultivated through a combination of physical postures, mindful breathing, and meditation. In the practice of yoga, individuals are encouraged to focus on the present moment, paying attention to their breath, sensations in the body, and the thoughts flowing through their minds.

- Mindful Movement (Asanas): The physical postures or asanas in yoga help individuals become aware of their bodies. As they move through different poses, practitioners develop a heightened sense of their muscles, joints, and overall physical sensations. This increased awareness extends beyond the mat and into daily life.
- Conscious Breathing (Pranayama): Yoga places a strong emphasis on conscious breathing or pranayama. By directing attention to the breath, individuals learn to control and deepen their breathing. This practice not only enhances lung capacity but also fosters mindfulness, as the breath becomes an anchor to the present moment.
- Meditation (Dhyana): Yoga often incorporates meditation techniques to quiet the mind and promote self-reflection. Regular meditation sessions allow individ-

uals to observe their thoughts without judgment, fostering a deep understanding of their inner world. This introspection contributes to increased self-awareness.

- Mind-Body Connection: Yoga encourages the integration of mind and body. Through the unity of physical postures, breath, and mental focus, practitioners develop awareness of the mind-body connection. This connection helps individuals to recognise how their mental and emotional states effects physically.
- Cultivation of Presence: The philosophy of yoga emphasises being present in the moment. As individuals engage in the practice, they learn to let go of distractions and concerns about the past or future. Being present is essential for building self-awareness, as it helps individuals focus on their current experiences.

In Thumbnail, self-awareness through yoga is a holistic process that involves integrating mindful movement, conscious breathing, meditation, and a heightened awareness of the mind-body connection. By regularly engaging in these practices, individuals can develop a profound understanding of themselves and their emotional states.

Where most of you fall short. You don't pay attention to your bodies until they break down and cry for help. To all the Mothers, Fathers, Students and Working professionals I would like to say: Prioritise yourself. Don't let push your body to the extent that it completely stops functioning. Remember "There is always a way-When you are committed" - Tony Robbins

You have to take out 45 minutes everyday.

To nurture your inner being by embracing self-care practices that promote healing.

To cultivate a positive mindset to sow the seeds of self-restoration and well-being.

To unearth the power within you to mend the wounds of the past and foster personal healing.

To embrace self-love as a balm for your soul.

To reconnect with your inner strength to rebuild, renew, and heal from life's challenges.

To embracing forgiveness.

You look for cures for diseases that can be simply avoided. Most lifestyle diseases are curable through yoga.

But they are also avoidable. If you had an option to either protect your money or retrieve it once it's stolen, you'd rather protect it. Right? Your body is the currency you have in the material world. Taking care of it to avoid any illness should be our primary concern. Instead of waiting for it to get sick, and to look for ways to cure it.

When yoga became part of my life, the challenges I faced with my body and mind didn't vanish overnight, but they slowly began to ease. It was a gradual journey—one that required time and patience—but it ended up transforming me in ways I could never have imagined. The time and effort I dedicated to my well-being eventually rewarded me with a stronger, healthier version of myself.

Many people start on their journey of health, focusing on just one aspect of themselves. To them I would like to say: imagine your body as a forest and a healthy lifestyle like an ecosystem that sustains that forest. The first question to ask yourself is: what makes up a forest? Is it just trees? No. Is it just animals? No. You cannot call just a group of trees or just a group of animals a forest. There are different elements, such as trees, animals, birds, mammals and some tiny microorganisms, algae, and insects that might not even come to your mind. The worms that burrow in the earth, the bugs that move from flower to flower carrying the pollens, and the fern on the trees, fungi and bacteria, they all come together to make a forest. Suppose you take away the bugs from this ecosystem. On the surface, it might not look like much, as bugs are so tiny. But the absence of even one set of organisms could have a tremendous effect. Without the bugs and bees, there won't be any way to carry out pollination. It would lead to fewer fruits and eventually no vegetation. Even the tiniest disturbance can send ripples through the entire forest, threatening its magical balance.

So, remember, every part, no matter how small, contributes to the harmony of your health forest.

Building a healthy lifestyle looks something similar. You are not just your body or your mind. Many people think that just exercising regularly can give them their goal of being healthy. Others might think that dieting can keep them fit. But exercising is like trees and dieting like animals. They might be the elements that you can see most clearly, however, there are many minute elements involved too. In reality, like an ecosystem, you have to incorporate a lot of habits and practices to keep yourself healthy. You cannot expect just one thing or the other to keep you healthy. You have to involve all parts of your life: your body, your mind, your food habits, sleeping cycle, gratitude practice, etc. Like different elements of a forest, these practices will come together naturally and build a healthy routine for you. It might not seem like a big deal to you, but even having your meals on time can have an immense effect on your body. This ecosystem of practices like Asanas (postures), Pranayam (Breathing Technique), Ahara (proper diet), and Nidra (proper sleeping routine) will ultimately heal you.

Building this ecosystem of healthy practices was a transformative journey for me. Let's say, Yoga is the trees for me, a healthy diet is the animals and birds, and a healthy sleep schedule is the insects. Small habits like having food on time, meditation, etc. are the Mammals. And the little aspects of the daily routine making my bed as soon as I wake up, lighting a lamp or praying to express my gratitude to the supreme are the pollens and microorganisms that work at the minute level, not visible to the naked eye, but extremely important.

I was at a low point in my life when I discovered Yoga. Once I became a Sadika (yoga practitioner) , all the other elements also came into my life naturally. Now, when I look at my life, I find it completely different from how it used to be. I now have my ecosystem to heal and sustain myself, and it all started on the yoga mat. But do you need to go through some disease or depression to turn to Yoga? No. The thing with lifestyle is, its a circle. There is no beginning, end, or middle. No point is a low point or high point. It's all part of your journey. You can get up right now and call it the starting point of your circle. You can take control of it regardless of where you are. After all, it's a circle, and only you know where you started.

But is it only women who can reap the benefits of yoga? NO, yoga is for everyone, regardless the age, gender, body type, religion, and anything you can think of. Men can experience a variety of stressors too, in both their work and family lives, and go through equally difficult life changes. Children as young as 8 years can have an overflow of energy in them, with anxiety and anger issues which can be very well handled through practicing yoga. The benefits of yoga for older adults are no less profound. From improving physical flexibility to enhancing mental clarity, managing chronic pain, and fostering emotional resilience, yoga has the power to transform the lives of older individuals. Its impact extends beyond the mat, reaching deep into the hearts and souls of those who practice it. You can consider yoga as a path to a healthier, more vibrant, and fulfilling future.

Here are some examples of why men should incorporate yoga into their daily lives and make it a lifestyle.

Take Aman, a 35-year-old marketing professional. Despite his success, he often feels unworthy and disconnected from himself. Yoga becomes his sanctuary. As he practices poses like Warrior II and Tree Pose, he discovers his inner strength and stability. The daily practice helps Aman embrace his imperfections and celebrate his unique journey.

Emotional resilience isn't just a skill; it's a necessity for navigating life's storms. Yoga offers men tools to manage their emotions, helping them process feelings rather than suppress them.

Rahul, a 29-year-old IT engineer, constantly battles work-related stress and burnout. Yoga introduces him to Pranayama (breathing exercises), which become his go-to remedy during tense moments. In poses like Child's Pose and Savasana, he finds the tranquility to process his worries. Each practice session leaves Rahul more equipped to handle life's pressures with grace.

For men, especially in an era dominated by screens and sedentary lifestyles, yoga serves as a gentle reminder of the synergy between the mind and body.

Vijay, a 40-year-old entrepreneur, had ignored his physical health for years, prioritizing work over wellness. Through yoga, he learns to listen to his body. Sun Salutations and core-strengthening poses rekindle his physical vitality, while mindfulness exercises deepen his mental clarity. This newfound connection empowers Vijay to lead a healthier, more intentional life.

Relationships thrive on empathy, respect, and balance. Yoga teaches men the value of these principles, fostering better connections in their personal and professional lives.

Arjun, a 25-year-old newlywed, struggled with balancing his marriage and career. Yoga classes with his partner became a bonding activity. Together, they practiced partner poses, which cultivated trust and communication. Off the mat, Arjun found himself more patient and understanding, enriching his relationships both at home and work.

Overall, practicing yoga can help men develop greater resilience and cope with stressors in both their work and family lives, leading to a greater sense of well-being and improved quality of life, and can see growth and prosperity in both.

Here are a few examples of why teens and undergrads should imbibe yoga in their lifestyle.

However, for teenagers and undergraduates, it takes on a special and vital role in their lives. It becomes not just a practice but a sanctuary, a guiding light, and a steadfast friend.

The Power of Self-Discovery:

During the tumultuous years of adolescence, young minds often find themselves adrift in a sea of uncertainty. It's a time when they grapple with identity, body changes, and the pressures of academic and social expectations. In this tempest, yoga serves as a lighthouse. It guides them toward self-discovery, helping them embrace their bodies and minds in a world that often tells them to be something they are not.

Consider Naira, a fourteen-year-old teen. She's shy, introverted, and struggling with self-esteem. The practice of yoga opens a door for her to explore her strengths and vulnerabilities. Through each asana, she learns to stand tall and breathe deep, not just on the mat but also in the face of life's challenges. With each class, she discovers the power of her body and the resilience of her spirit.

The Art of Emotional Resilience:

Emotions run deep during youth, and the rollercoaster of feelings can be overwhelming. Yoga provides a safe haven for teenagers and undergrads to understand and manage their emotions. It's a place where they learn to breathe through stress and be present in moments of joy.

Consider Shaurya, a seventeen-year-old high school student who is burdened with the weight of expectations from parents and peers. Yoga teaches him to find peace in the chaos. It is on the mat, in the depth of a pose, that he realises the art of letting go. Each exhalation becomes a release of pent-up frustration, and each inhales an infusion of renewed strength. Yoga helps Shaurya navigate the storms of his emotions, turning them into waves that he can ride with grace.

Strengthening the Mind-Body Connection:

In an age dominated by screens and distractions, the mind often becomes disconnected from the body. Yoga beautifully bridges this gap. It reminds teenagers and undergraduates that they are more than just their thoughts—they are a unified blend of body, mind, and spirit. Take Arpita, a twenty-year-old college student. Amidst lectures, assignments, and late-night study sessions, she often feels detached from his physical being. Yoga gently guides him back to his body. It teaches her that each stretch and twist is an act of self-love, and each breath is an acknowledgment of his existence. This newfound awareness transforms Arpita`s relationship with herself, helping her to better balance the demands of academic life.

Nurturing Healthy Relationships:

As young hearts begin to explore the complexities of relationships, yoga offers valuable lessons. It teaches the importance of respect, compassion, and empathy—values that are often overlooked in the frenetic pace of modern life.

Meet Hardeep, a sixteen-year-old who's learning about love and friendship. Yoga shows him that the same care he extends to himself on the mat can be offered to others. The sense of community and shared growth in a yoga class inspires him to cultivate healthier, more fulfilling relationships in him life outside the studio.

Yoga becomes a haven for teenagers and undergraduates, a timeless practice that weaves its emotional threads into their lives. It offers them the wisdom to stand tall in the face of adversity, the serenity to embrace their emotions, the awareness to unite mind and body, and the grace to nurture profound relationships. In every breath, every pose, and every moment of stillness, it whispers, "You are enough, just as you are."

Here is why women should embrace yoga in their lifestyle.

Yoga is a radiant gem that holds immense significance for women. It's not just a practice; it's a sanctuary where women can find empowerment, healing, and self-discovery. Let's explore why yoga is so important for women through the lens of personal stories and emotional experiences.

Empowerment through Strength:

Meet Shamita, a woman in her thirties who's juggling the responsibilities of work, family, and personal aspirations. Yoga becomes her sanctuary, a place where she can harness her physical strength and inner power. Through challenging poses, Shamita discovers that she's capable of so much more than she once believed. Her journey on the yoga mat mirrors her journey in life, teaching her that she can face challenges head-on and emerge stronger. The emotional transformation in her is palpable as she stands taller, both physically and metaphorically.

Emotional Resilience and Stress Relief:

For women dealing with the pressures of modern life, the emotional benefits of yoga are immeasurable. Take Janhvi, a young professional navigating a demanding career. The stresses of her job often threaten to overwhelm her. Through yoga, she finds solace and a way to release the emotional burdens she carries. The practice of mindfulness and deep breathing during yoga sessions helps her manage stress and anxiety. Janhvi`s emotional well-being is transformed as she learns to cultivate inner peace, resilience, and a calm mind, not just on the mat but in her daily life.

Healing from Within:

Yoga provides a profound avenue for emotional healing. Consider Richa, a survivor of a traumatic experience. The emotional scars run deep, and she finds it challenging to move forward. Through yoga, she embarks on a journey of self-compassion and healing. The gentle, nurturing poses and the emphasis on self-care become a sanctuary for her emotional recovery. She learns to release emotional pain, and her yoga mat becomes a space where she can mend her spirit. The transformation in her is profound as she moves from a place of hurt to one of healing.

Celebrating Self-Love and Acceptance:

In a world that often places unrealistic expectations on women, yoga becomes a refuge for self-love and acceptance. Women like Maanya, who have struggled with body image and self-esteem, find yoga to be a space for self-celebration. The practice of asanas teaches her to appreciate her body's strength and flexibility, regardless of its shape or size. Maanya`s emotional journey with yoga is one of embracing her uniqueness and cultivating self-love.

In the world of women, yoga is not just a physical practice; it's an emotional voyage. It is a place to discover and celebrate strength, find emotional resilience, heal from past wounds, and embrace self-love. It is where the mind, body, and soul unite in harmony, leading to a transformative emotional journey that empowers and uplifts women in a myriad of ways.

Here are a few examples of why senior citizens should include yoga in their lifestyle.

Fostering Flexibility and Stability With advancing years, the agility of the body often diminishes, making mundane activities a daunting endeavour. Yoga, with its gentle poses, acts as a balm, restoring elasticity and equilibrium. Ravi at 64, a septuagenarian grappling with stiff joints and wobbly footing, found solace in yoga. Through consistent engagement with poses like Downward Dog and Tree Pose, he reclaimed his physical grace. What was once a hesitant walk around the garden transformed into a confident morning stride.

Easing Persistent Aches and Pains The throes of chronic discomfort—be it arthritic agony or lingering backaches—are subdued through the mindful movements of yoga. Lakshmi, 68, who had long endured the tyranny of back pain, discovered liberation through poses like Sphinx and Cat-Cow. Each session reinforced her musculature, alleviating the strain on her spine and granting her a newfound sense of freedom.

Cultivating Inner Serenity Life's twilight years often amplify anxieties—health concerns, financial burdens, and solitude can shadow the mind. Yoga, with its rhythmic breathing techniques and meditative practices, dissolves such worries, instilling calm.

Ramesh at 63, a widower burdened by solitude, embraced the art of Pranayama. In the cadence of his breath, he unearthed solace, finding not only inner peace but also a renewed appreciation for the present.

Enhancing Cognitive Vitality Yoga fortifies the neural pathways, augmenting focus, memory, and mental acuity. When Sheela who is 61 years old notices a decline in her mental sharpness, integrated practices like alternate nostril breathing into her routine. Gradually, her memory sharpened, enabling her to actively partake in family discussions with vigour and joy.

Embracing Gratitude and Acceptance Yoga fosters an ethos of self-compassion and contentment, encouraging seniors to cherish the present and release past burdens. Manoj, a 75-year-old reflective of bygone regrets, found solace in yoga. The reflective moments during meditation became his refuge, teaching him to celebrate the simplicity of daily life.

Building Bonds Through Community Group yoga sessions cultivate a spirit of camaraderie, offering seniors a sanctuary to forge friendships and share experiences. Radha, 69, joined a community yoga class, where shared practice blossomed into shared laughter and stories, filling her days with companionship and joy.

Fortifying Independence and Self-Assurance

Yoga empowers seniors to maintain autonomy, fortifying their physical resilience and mental fortitude. Anita, at 80, feared becoming dependent on her children. Chair yoga introduced her to modified poses that strengthened her limbs, enabling her to tackle daily chores with newfound confidence.

But the question remains. What is yoga?

When you hear the word "yoga," the physical state of your body pops into your mind. All those complicated twisting of your limbs that seem almost impossible to achieve. You get riddled with the thoughts of your physical well-being, not being able to touch your toes without bending the knees, or that one time you sprained your lower back while doing the cobra pose. This train of thought is soon followed because you'll never find any time to practice yoga. Eventually, you shut down any thoughts of it, and go back to slouching in front of your laptop, sending out work emails. (Reminder: I see you slouching while reading this too. Fix your posture).

It's not your fault. We like to think we control our thoughts, but a lot of them are shaped by mass media. This is how trends work—they take something familiar, give it a fresh spin, and suddenly it feels brand new. The media plays a big role in this. It shows us what's popular, what we should pay attention to, and even how we should feel about it. Over time, these repeated messages shape our thoughts, preferences, and even our habits.

Take fashion trends, for example. A certain color or style becomes "must-have," and suddenly, you notice it everywhere. It's not that these things weren't around before, but once they're spotlighted by influencers, advertisements, or celebrities, they seem more appealing.

The same happens with our opinions and beliefs. We might think we've formed them independently, but in reality, they're often shaped by the media we consume. That's why it's important to step back sometimes, question what we see, and ask ourselves if we truly agree with it—or if we're just following the crowd.

But I digress. Our original concern remains that a vast majority of the population thinks of yoga as a physical endeavour. As kids, we've all challenged each other in school to see how far we could go in a leg split, how flexible our spine was, or if we could touch our head to our knees without bending the latter.

There are two major questions.

1. Is Yoga only about the physical lengths your body can reach?
2. Where did that child in you who was constantly trying to stretch the boundaries of his/her physical strength?

This image of yoga being a physical pursuit isn't necessarily wrong. A very small aspect of yoga is, in fact, all about the postures of the body. We call them Asanas. In simple terms, asanas are postures that a body takes. You may be sitting or lying down while reading this book. You're in an asana. When we feel alert, we sit up straight.

But is Yoga only for asanas?

Is Yoga Only About Asanas?

Asanas is one of the eight limbs (Ashtanga) of Yoga. The Ashtanga of Yoga was propagated by Sage Patanjali in his Yoga Sutras. In it, out of 196 sutras, only 3 of them speak of asanas directly. The eight limbs of yoga include Yama (moral codes), Niyama (self-discipline), Asana (posture), Pranayama (breath control), Pratyahara (sense withdrawal),

Dharana (concentration), Dhyana (meditation), and Samadhi (oneness with the self). Asana is just one of these. Yama is a responsibility or behaviour that the eight-limbed path of yoga recommends as a part of its philosophy and teaching. Niyamas refers to internal observances, or commitments to oneself.

Asanas is what comes to the mind of an average person when they think of Yoga. The complicated postures that make the body look boneless, is the image people have embedded in their minds. But the truth is, asanas are only a very minuscule part of the entirety of the experience that yoga offers. It only prepares you for what awaits you in your journey with Yoga ahead. The word 'yoga' has been derived from the Sanskrit root word of 'yuj' broadly meaning 'union'. In the second Sutra of the Samadhi Pada of the Yoga Sutras of Patanjali, Yoga is defined as 'Yogaha chitta vritti nirodhah'. It'll be a fantastical day when a given sentence can be translated without altering the meaning behind it. But to provide an essential translation, the definition in English would be "Yoga is to control the modification or the functioning of the mind'.

Nowhere in this definition is the body mentioned. Sure the mind is a part of the body, but if Yoga is so popularly known as a practice that cures bodily diseases then why does the most authoritative text on yoga define it with no mention of the word 'body'?

Now simplifying it.

Think of a new phone. It runs smoothly, loads the contents of an app quickly, you could be scrolling on instagram with a Netflix show running simultaneously and yet nothing will lag. Because the mind, therefore the memory, of the phone isn't filled with cache and automated downloads from different apps. Eventually, the local storage of your phone along with cloud storage gets cluttered with tiny insignificant files that you'll never look at again, good morning images from family members, love poems from your beloved, funny content from your friends and what not. Initially it's not much of a problem since your phone will lag only when you're making it do a lot of heavy lifting. But then it stops functioning while doing the most basic task it was made for doing. Calling, Texting and now for Making payments. That's when the real trouble begins. Then you're forced to go through those in-numerous files, delete them, reboot your phone just to make it capable of doing the simplest of tasks. Frustrating right? This is how most of us treat ourselves. The human child is much like a new phone. He/She doesn't tire out, runs explosively without stopping, learns many new life skills on an hourly basis, more often than not, especially in multilingual countries, like India picks up two languages at a time and is ever curious. But as you age, along with all the essential life skills. You also end up acquiring years of internalised trauma. This is a huge blow to your self-esteem. Your mind ends up in conflict with your body. It reaches a point where you feel completely disconnected from your own body.. You don't feel like challenging yourselves physically anymore. It's not because you are not capable. But because your normal life itself has become such a huge challenge that even the thought of further challenges makes your blood run cold. This is where your problem lies. It is because your mind is cluttered with unwelcoming thoughts, that your body lags in doing the most fundamental chores. Let's take the most essential chore of humans.

Sleep.

You can still go without food for a week, but sleep you simply cannot ignore. Every animal needs it. Even the plants sleep. When was the last time you went to bed on time or even had a long uninterrupted sleep daily in a row, for a month? The body restores and repairs itself during sleep, both physically and mentally, especially during uninterrupted sleep.

Those who don't get enough sleep, cannot work efficiently. You don't have to observe a yogi to see whether the body and mind really are connected. Such small examples from our daily routine serve as an excellent examples of how the mind and the body are correlated. A well rested mind helps the body perform better and a well rested body gives you a peaceful mind. A huge part of our population suffers from sleep related disorders, and most of the cases just go undiagnosed primarily because lack of sleep isn't necessarily considered unhealthy.

There's no popular "trend" or discourse around it. The issue here is, we have a vicious circle. The mind is disturbed because the body is unhealthy and the body is unhealthy because the mind is disturbed.

You can choose to start with either the mind or the body to improve this circle of lifestyle. The ultimate aim of Yoga is to achieve control over our minds. Time and again, you are reminded of a simple truth. It is easier to control your body than to gain the same level of control over your mind. This is why the most authoritative texts on Yoga emphasise starting with the body. They advise mastering asanas and pranayamas first. These practices are seen as steps toward achieving control over the mind. To sit down and meditate, requires an immense amount of inner peace and concentration. But it also requires the physical strength to sit up still and straight for an extended period of time. Yoga is a lifestyle. Asanas are simply one of the first steps towards achieving that lifestyle. The aim of yoga is to achieve the union of the mind and the body. Once this is achieved, the union of oneself with the universe is the step that follows.

Tracing The History of Yoga

In the Yogic lore, Shiva is the first Guru/Yogi and is known as Adiguru/Adiyogi. It is known that he imparted the knowledge of Yoga to the saptarishis or the seven sages. These sages, carrying this knowledge, travelled to the seven continents with the goal to disseminate this science of growing beyond the physical limitations of the human body and achieving higher forms of consciousness.

However, let's have a look at the definite traces of Yoga throughout the history of humankind.

Ancient Origins

Yoga found its earliest written documentation in the sacred scriptures known as the Vedas, which are approximately 10,000 years old.

The wisdom of sages was passed down through generations as an oral tradition, fostering the spiritual awakening of those who sought it.

Similarly, Buddhism, which emerged in India in the 5th century BCE, also has a rich tradition of yoga and meditation practices.

In fact, many of the asanas (postures) commonly associated with yoga today have their roots in Buddhist meditation practices.

8th century is period that was marked as the birth of the Upanishads. Upanishads shifted the focus of the religious teachings of the Vedas to see things critically through a lens of philosophy.

They explored the writings and threw light on the inaccessible information in the Vedas on Yoga. With the view of attaining the ultimate aim of yoga i.e. self-realization or enlightenment, the Upanishads elaborate on meditation and mantra recitations. 20 of the 108 Upanishads are dedicated to the techniques to be followed in the practice of Yoga like Pranayama for breath exercises to establish control over breathing.

Yoga took on various forms, from the meditative practices of Raja Yoga to the physical postures of Hatha Yoga. These practices were a means to unite the physical and spiritual aspects of the self, bringing individuals into a harmonious emotional balance with the world around them.

Overall, while the origins of yoga may be shrouded in some ambiguity, it is clear that this ancient practice has had a profound impact on Indian culture and spirituality, as well as on the wider world. Its continued popularity and relevance today is a testament to the enduring power and adaptability of this remarkable practice.

The Classical Period of Yoga (500 BCE - 800 CE)

During this time, key texts and teachings shaped the foundation of yoga. The Bhagavad Gita, the Yoga Sutras of Sage

Patanjali, and the teachings of Lord Buddha and Lord Mahavir emerged. Lord Mahavir emphasized meditation, while Lord Buddha introduced specific postures for enlightenment. This period highlighted the role of the mind in yoga and developed the concept of Yoga sadhana as a path to spiritual growth.

This period gave to the world the Bhagavad Gita. A symbolic dialogue between Lord Krishna (Universal Consciousness) and Prince Arjuna (Human Consciousness) where we find the first mention of the three spiritual paths: Karma Yoga i.e. the path of unselfish action; Bhakti Yoga i.e. the path of dedicated and loving actions; Gnana Yoga i.e. the path of knowledge. Lord Krishna, in a very succinct manner, summaries what 'Yoga' means by saying "Samatvam Yoga Uchyate" i.e. maintaining an equilibrium of the mind or remaining centered in any given situation, whether adverse or favourable, joyous or upsetting, is Yoga.

In the 2nd BCE Maharishi Patanjali, also known as the father of Yoga, wrote and compiled the Yoga Sutras, the first document that systematised the study and practice of Yoga. The yoga in these sutras came to be called Raja Yoga. It is in the Yoga Sutras that we find the Ashtanga Yoga or the eight limbs of yoga i.e.

1. Yama or External Disciplines
2. Niyama or Internal Disciplines
3. Asana or Postures
4. Pranayama or Breathing Exercises
5. Pratyahara or Withdrawal of Senses
6. Dharana or Concentration
7. Dhyana or Meditative Absorption

8. Samadhi or Union, Integration

In the modern times, we have five spiritual paths to yoga. The first three came from the Bhagavad Gita (Karma, Bhakti, Jnana), the fourth one from the Yoga Sutras(Raja Yoga) and the fifth one from The Hatha Yoga Pradipika (Hatha Yoga).

Patanjali's Yoga Sutra was heavily referenced by its contemporaneous texts. The Mahabharata mentions certain terms explained in the Yoga Sutras like Vichara (subtle reflection) and Viveka (discretion). It also mentions the crux of what Yoga offers. The separation of the soul from the material world and the amalgamation of the former with the universe. Similarly, mudras mentioned in the Yoga Sutra are referenced in the Natya Shastra. Ved Vyas' commentary on the Yoga Sutras expounds on the relationship between the Yoga School, relating to meditation and contemplation, and the Samkhya School, relating to consciousness and matter, of the Hindu Philosophy.

The Period of Shankaracharya and Tulsidas (Post Classical Period)

This period brought sages like Adi Shankaracharya who added to the existing teachings and techniques of Raj and Jnana Yoga, of which the techniques and yogic rituals of the latter can help achieve Nirvana. This period also saw the rise of Tulsidas and Purnadaradasa Much like the Classical period, meditation and the mind was emphasised, however, the highlight of this period was the practice of Hatha Yoga.

- This period is the closest to the interpretation of what we perceive Yoga to be. Characterised by the importance of physical well-being, the period brought forth renowned yogis like

- Swami Vivekananda,
- Ramana Maharishi,
- BKS Iyengar,
- K Pattabhi Jois,
- Paramhansa Yogananda.

The modern period marked a crucial turning point in the history of Yoga. Swami Vivekananda opened the eyes of the world to the science of Yoga. In the late 19th century he visited the United States, originally as a delegate to the World's Parliament of Religions, where he delivered his historic speech on inter religious tolerance. His next few years were spent touring the USA, imparting the knowledge of Yoga in the West. His speeches and translations of Sanskrit works of Yoga into English laid the groundwork for the spread of Yoga by his contemporary yogis and gurus in the West.

While in the post classical period, the mind and the physical body were given equal importance, in the modern period the focus slightly shifted from the balance of both the mind and the body to mostly the body. This brings us to another extremely pressing issue that the community of Yoga instructors are facing today. This shift of focus of yoga from the mind to the body has put a pressure to innovate, rebrand and repackage Yoga into something that is far from what it was originally supposed to be.

The Pressure to Innovate

We've all read this somewhere or the other, "Capitalism breeds innovation." But there's hardly any discourse around the pressure to innovate, and the consequences of such innovations. A lot many things are invented for one purpose or the other, but over the years, become a victim to evolution, eventually losing the essential purpose they were made for. If you ever find the time, I'd suggest you go through the illustrious history of Listerine, the mouthwash found in every household. It started off as a surgical antiseptic, in 1888 an ad claimed Listerine to be able to cure sweaty feet, corns between the toes, later on it was advertised as a refreshing additive to cigarettes, an ailment for the flu and a treatment for dandruff. Other such products would be Coca Cola, originally produced as a soft alternative for people with morphine addiction, mild headache and anxiety. The rest is history. A computer virus was invented only to see how an unwanted file would affect the system. Again, the rest is history.

In a free market economy, everything you offer becomes a commodity. But the crucial ingredient is, you must know how to convince people to use that commodity. In this day and age of information and marketing, as mentioned before, a lot gets lost in 'trends'. Nobody wishes to truly understand the fundamentals of what is being offered to them.

We live in a world of instant gratification that is driven more by the results of something rather than the process of it. We're surrounded by click-baits and claims that project an incredible result within a short period of time. These clickbait articles and video tutorials like "Abs in just two weeks?" "Say goodbye to those hip dips" are one of the few examples of how the fitness community is struggling to cater to the demand of the public. RESULTS.

This is where all the trouble begins. What people fail to understand is that the human body isn't made to mindlessly workout in reps of 10 x 4. Focusing only on the body while leaving the mind behind to its own devices is almost just as detrimental to the holistic health of an individual. Sure your muscles may pop out in just 2 weeks as promised, but it will most likely be at the cost of a mental and physical burnout. The mind is just as much a part of your body as your muscles are and should be taken care of equally. This is why Yoga, in the past few years, Specially post covid has become a popular choice, because it offers to work on the mind and the body and the soul.

However, a fair amount of Yoga instructors I have personally spoken to, have admitted of facing a similar issue of being under the pressure to innovate and reinvent Yoga. The fact that two years of covid lockdown period saw an intense rise in the number of people turning to yoga. But it doesn't help much either since the geographical limit of admitting students became non-existent. The world was now not limited to offline yoga classes available in their neighborhood. You could be sitting in Germany and could enroll yourself in an online course offered by a CertifiedYoga Master in India. While there was a fair amount of competition even before, this kind of accessibility to yoga Masters online led to a rise in competition between Yoga Masters, Yoga Therapist, Yoga Instructors etc and what they offered. Naturally, whatever they offered had to be significantly different from the other offers.

While a little rebranding hasn't hurt anyone, the extent to which Yoga Masters have to innovate and reinvent to grab the attention of their students and algorithm of various social media platforms is threatening to undermine the original essence of Yoga. It doesn't matter if you start off with the techniques of Raja Yoga or Jnana Yoga, the path should always lead to the realisation of the self. Again, whether or not you reach such a stage is immaterial, but you must be on the right path i.e. the path to self realisation or enlightenment or nirvana or whatever name you would like to give it.

Preserving the essence of yoga in the modern world is like safeguarding a precious gem against the tides of time. As we navigate our fast-paced, technology-driven lives, it's essential to keep the spiritual and philosophical roots of yoga alive.

Meditation is as significant as Asanas: In a world filled with distractions, embrace meditation. Take time to meditate, be present in the moment, and connect with your inner self. Yoga's essence lies in self-awareness and introspection.

Honour Tradition: Respect the wisdom of ancient yogic texts and teachings. Delve into the ancient scriptures and understand the philosophical underpinnings that make yoga a holistic discipline.

Incorporate Yoga Philosophy: Integrate the yamas and niyamas (moral and ethical principles) into your daily life. Living by these principles, such as non-violence (ahimsa) and self-discipline (tapas), helps maintain the spiritual core of yoga.

Practice Yoga as a lifestyle: Adapt your yoga practice to suit your modern life. While honouring tradition is vital, customise your routine to address your specific physical, mental, and emotional needs.

Cultivate Compassion: Embody compassion not only towards others but also towards yourself. Yoga's essence lies in fostering love and understanding, both for the world around you and your own inner self.

Balance Technology: While technology can be a source of distraction, it can also aid your yoga journey. Use apps and online resources to connect with the global yoga community and enhance your practice.

Eco-Friendly Living: Embrace eco-conscious living, respecting the environment. Yoga and sustainability go hand in hand, as they both signify a deeper connection with the world we inhabit.

Keep Learning: Stay open to learning and growth. The essence of yoga lies in continuous self-improvement. Attend workshops, read books, and seek guidance to deepen your understanding of yourself.

In this modern age, where the pace of life seems relentless, it is our duty to preserve the essence of yoga. By nurturing the spiritual, philosophical, and ethical aspects, we can ensure that yoga remains a guiding light on our journey towards self-discovery and well-being.

Research on the Benefits of Yoga

Over the years, many curious physiologists, psychologists and scientists have dipped their toes into researching the effects of Yoga on various systems of the body and on the overall quality of life of someone who practices Yoga. In the later chapters, system specific researches are discussed, but here let's have a look at some of the leading research done on lifestyle changes that yoga offers.

Immunity

Over the course of the past 4 years of Covid-19, the word immunity has been thrown around so casually that most of us have become immune to it. However, a good immune system is indispensable to surviving unprecedented medical challenges like Covid-19. William Bushell, PhD, MIT, led a comprehensive review of over a hundred scientific studies done on yoga and immunity. A number of scientific findings in the review showed anti-inflammatory and anti stress properties of yoga practices. The findings indicated that meditation and yoga practices increase the vagal tone[1]. Vagal tone is one of the most basic components of the parasympathetic nervous system and an increased vagal tone could help the body relax or recover faster after having experienced stress[2].

In a paper, done by researchers from the Massachusetts Institute of Technology, University of California-San Diego, Chopra Library for Integrative Studies, and Harvard University, experts explain the benefits that yoga and meditation may have as an adjunctive treatment to the novel coronavirus.

Anxiety

Anxiety is one of those baneful experiences we've all gone through at least once in our lifetime. For some it comes only before an exam or before going on stage while for the less fortunate ones it is a part of their daily routine. "What if I couldn't calculate the exact change that the shopkeeper has to return to me?" or "What if everyone stares at me if, I enter late in the classroom?" or "What if I mispronounce a word in front of my friends?". This is what the mind of an anxious person looks like, for the better part of their lives. Apart from being a condition in itself, anxiety is also a symptom for many other conditions like panic disorder, post traumatic stress disorder, social anxiety disorder, phobias etc. Those who go through this, know how much time they could save for themselves if only they didn't experience anxiety.

A study done in 2016[3] shows that the subjects who showed high levels of anxiety at the beginning of the study benefited the most from Hatha yoga.

Another study done in 2010 [4] compared the effects of yoga as opposed to walking. It showed how the increase in GABA(gamma aminobutyric acid) levels improved the mood and anxiety of those who practiced yoga.

Stress

Another pressing condition that disrupts the lifestyle of a significant part of the population. Whether it's adults or school-going kids, stress levels have risen significantly in recent years. Anxiety can be a symptom of many disorders. Stress, on the other hand, can be a cause of several issues. It can lead to cardiovascular problems and lower immunity. It can worsen conditions like asthma, depression, and anxiety. The list goes on..

A study done in 2016[5] took 70 participants within the age bracket of 35-60 years who were suffering from chronic periodontitis. Previously studies had shown that psychological stress among others were associated with this disease and its progression along with its healing. The 70 subjects were split into 3 groups. Group I included people suffering from stress, Group II included people without stress, Group III included people who had already been practicing yoga. The study showed that serum cortisol levels were higher in subjects from Group I when compared to Group II and III. Group III which consisted of the subjects that practiced yoga showed optimum levels of cortisol. Stress can cause a surge in cortisol levels which in turn damages blood vessels and causes an increase in blood pressure. This study's findings indicated that the group that had been practicing yoga had lower cortisol levels.

Yoga has been recognised by The National Institute of Health of the USA as a form of Complementary and Alternative Medicine. It offers a holistic lifestyle change. Where one problem, which is tied to several others, gets treated in a manner that the other issues dissipate along with it. Discussed above are 3 such issues. Anxiety, stress and immunity. In being able to treat these issues, a number of other medical conditions become manageable, or easier to treat, since anxiety, stress and low immunity levels provide a lot of friction and tend to work against any treatment for an ailment.

Thus, various research and studies have recognised and provided a scientific explanation of the age-old practice of Yoga. Even though it didn't need the stamp of approval, however, now that the whole world recognises the benefits of Yoga, it's time for more and more people to learn and apply it in their lives. This book will not only guide you through understanding what Yoga is, but also how to make it a part of your life and achieve your dream of living a healthy lifestyle.

References

[1] https://www.yogajournal.com/yoga-101/strength-your-immune-system-with-yoga/

[2]https://sass.uottawa.ca/sites/sass.uottawa.ca/files/how_to_stimulate_your_vagus_nerve_for_better_mental_health_1.pdf

[3] Hofmann SG, Andreoli G, Carpenter JK, Curtiss J. Effect of Hatha Yoga on Anxiety: A Meta-Analysis. J Evid Based Med. 2016;9(3):116-124. doi:10.1111/jebm.12204

[4]Streeter CC, Whitfield TH, Owen L, et al. Effects of yoga versus walking on mood, anxiety, and brain GABA levels: a randomized controlled MRS study. J Altern Complement Med. 2010;16(11):1145-1152. doi:10.1089/acm.2010.0007

[5] Katuri KK, Dasari AB, Kurapati S, Vinnakota NR, Bollepalli AC, Dhulipalla R. Association of yoga practice and serum cortisol levels in chronic periodontitis patients with stress-related anxiety and depression. J Int Soc Prev Community Dent. 2016;6(1):7-14. doi:10.4103/2231-0762.175404

https://www.theladders.com/career-advice/yoga-meditation-coronavirus-treatment

Chapter 2
Transform Your Life with Yoga: Key Benefits Unveiled

Have you ever gone into something anticipating the worst and walked away with the most? Consider creating a fixed deposit and receiving the highest conceivable interest rate; purchasing a house but receiving a palace at the same price, or planting a tree and reaping the greatest abundance of fruit in your neighbourhood. How do you feel about that? Although such circumstances are uncommon, having your expectations realised and exceeded beyond your expectations is never a negative thing. Many people have found yoga to be a very gratifying experience. It's like making an investment in your soul's never-ending inner reservoir. If you do it every day, you will be able to access the vast number of resources that are already dormant within you.

People in today's environment vastly misunderstand the relevance of holistic wellness vs monetary affluence.

We now live a life devoted solely to work, yet as much time as it consumes, it also necessitates that we take better care of our mental, physical, and spiritual health. As discussed in the previous chapter, many people begin practising yoga in order to improve their physical fitness and flexibility in order to adapt to the fast-paced lifestyle that we now live. But yoga is more than just a workout. When done correctly and with dedication, it has the longest-lasting effects of any gym activity or diet. There's impressive research that shows many practitioners of yoga who got into it mainly for physical fitness realised that it changed their behaviour. In terms of thinking pattern. Which completely, shifted their motivation for practising yoga.

Workplaces are beginning to acknowledge the significance of holistic wellness for their employees. Companies are incorporating wellness programs that include yoga sessions, mindfulness workshops, and healthy eating initiatives. These programs not only enhance employee's health and productivity but also create a more positive and supportive work environment.

Education systems are also recognising the value of holistic wellness. Schools are introducing mindfulness and yoga programs to help students manage stress, improve focus, and develop emotional resilience. These initiatives equip young people with the tools they need to navigate the challenges of modern life and build a strong foundation for their future well-being.

In conclusion, while monetary affluence can provide comfort and security, it is holistic wellness that truly enriches our lives. Embracing practices like yoga can lead to profound changes in how we live, think, and interact with the world around us. By valuing and pursuing holistic wellness. we can achieve a more balanced, fulfilling, and purposeful existence.

Ancient Science or Myth

You must have heard that the benefits of yoga are endless, but people still hesitate to believe in it as an actual science. In the previous chapter, you learnt how one doesn't have to belong to a certain religion in order to practise yoga. The foundations of Yoga are based upon the ancient scientific systems that developed in the Bharat. If you delve just a little deeper, you will find many instances of modern science taking valuable inputs from ancient scientific systems to gain deeper insights about the world around us in the present day.

A report 2021 year revealed that NASA scientists have been using the Hindu Calendar's 'Panchaang' to predict various astronomical events like solar and lunar eclipses. Even if the news is false and fake, don't you know that even before NASA our religious gurus where referring to Panchang for thousands of years to celebrate festivals according to astronomy. The festivals that we celebrate are not accordance with the fixed date but the reputation of astronomical events in the sky. This is one of many texts written by the Rishis which where scientific in nature and high in accuracy.

Yajna Research

Making offerings into a consecrated fire is another important Sanskritic tradition of Yajna or Havan. It has been the subject of a lot of research in recent times to prove its unprecedented effects on one's health and environment. Research conducted in the field of allopathic medicine showed that no bacteria were killed when 1 kg of mango wood was burnt in a closed room, but when the same was burnt with Havan samagri, the bacterial count was reduced by 94%. The research also mentioned that Havan has shown results in reducing blood sugar levels and diabetes when done with appropriate samagri (ingredients) and suitable surroundings. It has also been said to increase the soil fertility of the environment wherever it is practised regularly.

There is an array of modern research that has been conducted on the ancient sciences of yogic rituals and traditions. As individuals of the twenty-first century, most of us consider only the western standards of research to prove a study is scientific enough. Whereas many of us fail to see the seriousness of ancient yogic traditions, the old scriptures have already described such traditions as a major part of a scientific system.

Yoga can be appropriately referred to as the science of unlimited human possibilities since, it allows us to fully express our innate potential. At the same time, yoga addresses all areas of conscious evolution's theory, psychology, and pragmatism at the same time. It does not solely aim to cure and prevent diseases by building physical strength, but it helps us re-integrate our consciousness with the "whole" through mental vigour and emotional resilience.

The Yoga Sutras of Patanjali are explicit in that the focus of the work is on the mind, also called chitta, or consciousness. This is both a simple and complex object and subject. The first sutra, "atha yognusanam" can be translated as: Now commence the discipline of re-integration. The idea here is about connecting the mind and body and finding unity with something greater than yourself. The first sutra can be understood like this: after you've done everything in life—studying, building a career, socialising, fulfilling duties, and taking care of responsibilities—there comes a moment when you feel a deep need to know yourself.

When your mind, body, and soul come together and say, "Now it's time for yoga," it's a special turning point. Interestingly, the first line of the book begins with the word "Now," which feels like it's left open on purpose.

Maharishi Patanjali chose this approach carefully. It's meant to make you realize that you've arrived at an important moment in your life and to give you the freedom to start this journey of self-discovery when you're ready.

Benefits of the Yogic Lifestyle

Now that you understand that yoga is much more than a ritualistic tradition or a fitness regimen, let's look at the different types of practices that fall under it. Yoga is an old tradition that integrates physical, mental, and spiritual ideals in order to elevate humanity. Maharishi Patanjali, India's great sage, defined the eightfold method of yoga in his famous Yoga Sutra, namely yama, niyama, asana, pranayama, pratyahara, dharna, dhyana, and samadhi. These practices are a vital aspect of the yogic lifestyle and are founded on ancient sciences that have been shown to have exceptional outcomes for health and the environment, some of which are mentioned below.

1. YAMA: Yama, the first of yoga's eight limbs, is concerned with one's ethical standards and sense of integrity, focusing on our actions and how we conduct ourselves in life. Yamas are universal behaviours that are most closely related to the Golden Rule, which states, "Do unto others as you would have them do unto you." It encourages us to treat others in the same way we would like to be treated.

For example, if you value kindness, respect, and fairness, you should extend those qualities to others in your actions and words. The idea promotes empathy by putting yourself in someone else's position, considering how your behaviour might affect them, and acting with compassion and understanding.

There are five yamas – Ahimsa (non-violence), Satya (truthfulness), Asteya (non-stealing), Brahmacharya (continence), and Aparigraha (non-covetousness).

2. NIYAMA: The second limb, Niyama, is concerned with self-discipline and spiritual observances. Attending temple or place of worship on a regular basis, paying gratitude before meals, practice meditation on daily basis, or taking contemplative walks alone are all instances of niyamas in action.

   There are five niyama – Saucha (cleanliness), Samtosa (contentment), Tapas (heat; spiritual austerities), Svadhyaya (study of the sacred scriptures and of one's self), and Isvara Pranidhana (surrender to God).

3. ASANA: Asanas, or yoga postures, are the third of the eight limbs of yoga. According to the yogic viewpoint, the body is a temple of the soul, and its maintenance is a crucial step in our spiritual development. We build the habit of discipline and the ability to concentrate via the practise of asanas, both of which are required for meditation.

4. PRANAYAMA: This fourth stage, which translates as "breath control," consists of practises aimed to achieve mastery over the respiratory process while recognising the link between the breath, the mind, and the emotions. As the English meaning of

pranayama, "life force extension," implies, yogis believe it not only rejuvenates the body but also extends life. Pranayama can be practised as an isolated technique (sitting and completing a series of breathing exercises) or as part of your daily hatha yoga regimen.

5. PRATYAHARA: The fifth of the eight limbs of yoga, pratyahara, denotes withdrawal or sensory transcendence. During this stage, we make a conscious effort to shift our attention away from the outer world and its stimuli. We direct our attention internally, acutely aware of, but detached from, our senses. Pratyahara practise allows us to take a step back and examine ourselves. This practice helps us notice our habits and cravings without reacting to them. For instance, if you crave a snack even when you're not hungry, pratyahara helps you recognise this craving without giving in to it. By doing this, we can see which behaviours might be harmful to our health and stop them from affecting our inner growth.

By regularly practicing pratyahara, we develop the ability to observe our thoughts and actions more objectively. For example, if you often feel the urge to check your phone every few minutes, pratyahara helps you notice this habit and understand why you do it. You might realise that it's just a way to avoid boredom or anxiety.

Once we identify these patterns, we can start making conscious choices to change them. Instead of automatically reaching for your phone, you might choose to take a deep breath and relax, or focus on a task at hand. This helps break the cycle of automatic behaviours and brings more mindfulness into our daily lives.

Pratyahara also enhances our ability to focus and concentrate. When we withdraw our senses from external distractions, we create a quiet space within ourselves. This inner quiet allows us to concentrate better on whatever we are doing, whether it's studying, working, or even just relaxing.

Imagine you're studying for an important exam. Normally, you might get distracted by noises around you, like people talking or cars honking. With pratyahara, you train yourself to remain focused on your studies despite these distractions. Over time, this practice can improve your ability to concentrate and make you more productive.

In essence, pratyahara helps us gain control over our senses and impulses. It teaches us to respond thoughtfully rather than react impulsively. This control leads to a calmer, more centered mind, which is essential for deeper stages of meditation and self-awareness.

Overall, pratyahara is a powerful tool for self-improvement. By turning our attention inward and observing our thoughts and behaviours without judgment. You can make positive changes that enhance our physical, mental, and emotional well-being. It helps you live more mindfully, making better choices that support your health and inner growth.

6. DHARANA: Practicing pratyahara sets the stage for dharana, which means concentration. Each stage of yoga prepares you for the next one. After learning to withdraw from the distractions of the outside world,. You can now focus on dealing with the distractions of our mind. This isn't easy!

In dharana, you learn to slow down your thoughts by focusing on a single mental object. For example, you might focus on an energetic center in your body, like your heart or forehead. Or you might visualise an image of a deity or repeat a mantra silently in your mind.

Before reaching this stage, you have already started to develop your focus through the earlier steps: posture (asana), breath control (pranayama), and sensory withdrawal (pratyahara). For instance, in asana, holding a pose requires concentration. In pranayama, controlling the breath requires you to focus on your breathing pattern. In pratyahara, you practice ignoring external distractions.

In dharana, you take this focus to the next level by fixing your attention on one specific point. Imagine staring at a candle flame without letting your mind wander. Or repeating a calming word, like "peace," over and over in your head. This intense focus helps to quiet the mind.

As you practice concentrating for longer periods, it naturally leads to meditation (dhyana). For example, if you can concentrate on your breath for several minutes without getting distracted, you'll find it easier to enter a meditative state. Meditation is when this focused concentration becomes effortless and continuous.

Dharana builds on the skills developed in the previous stages. By learning to concentrate on a single point, you prepare yourselves for deeper meditation, where your mind becomes completely absorbed and quiet. This progression helps you achieve greater mental clarity and inner peace.

As you continue to practice dharana, you'll notice improvements in your ability to concentrate on tasks in your daily life. For instance, if you're working on a project, you might find it easier to stay focused without getting distracted by emails or phone notifications. This enhanced concentration can lead to greater productivity and a deeper sense of accomplishment.

Furthermore, dharana helps in managing stress and anxiety. By training your mind to focus on one thing at a time, you reduce the tendency to overthink or worry about multiple issues simultaneously. For example, if you're feeling overwhelmed by numerous tasks, practicing dharana can help you concentrate on just one task, reducing stress and making the workload feel more manageable.

Incorporating dharana into your daily routine can be simple. You can start with short sessions of focused concentration and gradually increase the duration as you become more comfortable. For example, you might begin with five minutes of focusing on your breath each morning. Over time, you can extend this practice to longer periods and explore other focal points like a mantra or a visual object.

In addition to improving mental clarity, dharana can also enhance emotional well-being. When you focus on positive mental objects, like a serene landscape or a beloved mantra, it can uplift your mood and foster a sense of inner calm. For example, visualising a peaceful beach scene can transport your mind to a place of tranquility, reducing feelings of anxiety or sadness.

As dharana becomes a regular practice, it sets a solid foundation for meditation (dhyana). In dhyana, the focus becomes so profound that there is a seamless flow of concentration, leading to a state of deep meditation. This state brings about profound insights, emotional healing, and a deeper connection to one's inner self.

In conclusion, dharana is a crucial step in the journey of yoga. By practicing dharana, you can enhance your concentration, reduce stress, improve emotional well-being, and pave the way for a more mindful and fulfilling life.

1. DHYANA: The seventh step of ashtanga yoga is meditation, or contemplation, known as dhyana. This stage involves an uninterrupted flow of focus. While concentration (dharana) and meditation (dhyana) might seem similar, there's a subtle difference between them. Dharana is about focusing on one thing at a time, like staring at a candle flame or repeating a mantra. In contrast, dhyana is being deeply aware without focusing on anything specific. At this point, the mind is quiet and produces few or no thoughts, creating a sense of profound calm.

Reaching this state requires significant strength and endurance. Imagine sitting still and quieting your mind completely for an extended period—this can be challenging! However, don't get discouraged. Yoga is a journey, and every step offers benefits, even if you don't achieve the "perfect" posture or state of consciousness.

For instance, when you practice dharana by focusing on your breath, you might initially struggle to keep your mind from wandering. Over time, as you get better at this, you might find moments where your mind becomes naturally quiet and still. These moments are glimpses of dhyana.

Another example is when you're deeply engrossed in an activity you love, such as painting or playing music. You might find yourself so absorbed that time seems to disappear, and your mind feels calm and clear. This experience is similar to dhyana, where awareness flows effortlessly without conscious effort.

Remember, the goal is not to force your mind into silence but to cultivate a practice that gradually leads to this state. Each time you sit to meditate, whether you achieve deep stillness or not, you're making progress. It's like training for a marathon—each run builds your stamina, even if you don't run the full distance every time.

In conclusion, dhyana is a state of deep, effortless awareness that follows concentration. While it requires practice and patience to achieve, the journey itself is rewarding. Every step you take in your yoga practice brings you closer to inner peace and clarity, demonstrating that the process is just as valuable as the goal.

2. SAMADHI: Samadhi, the eighth and final stage of ashtanga yoga, is a state of bliss. In this stage, the meditator merges completely with their focus and transcends the Self entirely. This experience leads to a profound connection with the Divine and a deep sense of interconnection with all living things. The result is a "peace that surpasses all understanding," a feeling of joy and unity with the Universe.

To some, this might sound like a lofty, almost unattainable goal. But let's break it down with examples.

Imagine a musician who becomes so absorbed in playing their instrument that they lose all sense of time and self. They are fully present in the music, feeling a deep connection to the notes, the rhythm, and the audience. This is similar to the experience of samadhi, where the meditator is fully immersed in their practice and experiences a profound sense of unity.

Another example is an athlete who enters the "zone" during a game. They perform at their peak, feeling a seamless connection between their mind and body. They are so focused that they move effortlessly and intuitively. This state of flow is akin to samadhi, where the meditator experiences a complete merging with their focus and a transcendence of the self.

A more everyday example could be a gardener who finds immense joy and peace while tending to their plants. He feels connected to the earth, the plants, and the cycles of nature. This deep connection and contentment reflect the blissful state of samadhi, where one feels a part of something much larger and more profound.

Samadhi is not about being "holier than thou" but about reaching a state of inner peace and connection that is possible for anyone with dedicated practice. It's the culmination of the journey through the stages of yoga, where each step prepares the meditator for this ultimate experience of unity and bliss.

Samadhi also brings a sense of equanimity. In the face of challenges and difficulties, a person who has experienced samadhi remains calm and composed. They see beyond the immediate situation and understand their place within the larger context of life. This perspective allows them to navigate life's ups and downs with grace and resilience.

For instance, a surgeon performing a complex operation might enter a state of deep focus and calm, aware of every movement and decision but not overwhelmed by the pressure of the situation. This focused calm can be seen as a high state of awareness, where the surgeon's skill, concentration, and sense of purpose come together in a moment of profound effectiveness and peace.

In essence, samadhi is not an escape from reality but a deeper engagement with it. It is the realisation of our deepest potential and our most profound connections. It is a state of being where we experience life with clarity, joy, and a sense of unity with all that is. While it is the final stage of the ashtanga path, its benefits permeate every aspect of our lives, transforming our everyday experiences into opportunities for profound peace and fulfilment.

Samadhi is a state of profound bliss and unity, where the meditator transcends the self and connects deeply with the Divine and all living things. While it may seem like an idealistic goal, examples from everyday life show that moments of deep immersion, flow, and connection are accessible to us all, demonstrating the potential for experiencing samadhi.

Yogic Lifestyle and Covid in India

The growth of COVID-19 and the tragedy we all experienced over the last few years compelled many of us to seek answers. Many people sensed the urgent necessity for a course adjustment to ensure human survival. This prompted numerous questions in our knowledge base and the associated societal and individual ways of living.

The lockdown and social isolation resulted in difficulties such as stress, worry, fear, loneliness, sadness, impatience, insomnia, disorientation, anger, frustration, and boredom. Moreover, the increasing incidence of COVID-19 cases and deaths heightened people's tension and anxiety. While scientists were busy finding cures for the Coronavirus, the masses were strongly advised to work on building up the body's immunity level. Almost all health practitioners, regardless of their field, emphasised the importance of having a strong immune system.

In response to the pandemic, many people turned to various methods to enhance their immunity. These included dietary changes, exercise, and adopting new wellness practices such as yoga and meditation. The focus on immunity became a central theme in health discussions. Experts were recommending a balanced diet rich in vitamins and minerals, regular physical activity, adequate sleep, and stress management techniques.

For example, people were encouraged to consume foods high in vitamin C, such as citrus fruits, and vitamin D, which can be obtained from sunlight or supplements. Regular exercise, such as walking, running, or home workouts, was promoted to keep the body active and strengthen the immune system. Mindfulness practices, such as meditation and yoga, were recommended to help manage stress and improve overall mental well-being.

Social support networks also played a crucial role during this time. Virtual gatherings, online support groups, and tele-health consultations became vital tools for maintaining social connections and accessing mental health resources. These measures helped individuals cope with the emotional and psychological challenges brought about by the pandemic.

The pandemic also highlighted the importance of public health measures and personal responsibility in preventing the spread of infectious diseases. Wearing masks, practicing social distancing, and frequent hand-washing became part of the new normal. These actions, combined with vaccination efforts, were essential in controlling the spread of the virus and protecting vulnerable populations.

In conclusion, the COVID-19 pandemic underscored the critical importance of building and maintaining a robust immune system. It brought to light the interconnectedness of physical, mental, and emotional health and the need for a holistic approach to well-being. By focusing on immunity and adopting healthier lifestyles, individuals can better prepare themselves for future health challenges.

The immunity of the host is an essential requisite to facilitate the eradication of infections. Disturbed immune systems seen as lymphopenia and elevated C-reactive protein levels are recognised to be the characteristic features in severely affected cases of COVID-19 infection. Extensive work has shown that systematic special tailor-made asana practices, dedicated pranayamas, meditation, and mantras could provide a broad-spectrum immune build up in the body so that viral infection could be averted and/or its virulence reduced.

After witnessing the impact of increasing Coronavirus, Honourable Prime Minister, Narendra Modi, advocated Yoga and requested that the Ayush Ministry follow the rules. He spoke during a session commemorating the 7th International Yoga Day, where he also discussed the M-Yoga application developed in conjunction with the World Health Organization (WHO). Mr. Modi stated that yoga has arisen as a force for unity that transcends race, colour, gender, creed, and nations. "Yoga contributes to our quest for a healthy planet." It has evolved as a force for togetherness that strengthens human relationships. It makes no distinctions. It transcends race, colour, gender, faith, and nation. Yoga is accessible to everyone." Prime Minister Narendra Modi termed yoga a "ray of hope" and a source of strength in the midst of the coronavirus pandemic. Yoga became a source of inner strength among people amid the novel coronavirus pandemic in India. It inculcated a faith in them that they could fight the virus.

Yoga has widely emerged as a form of public health support during the pandemic. Before the COVID-19 pandemic, yoga has been used in different social contexts, from small groups to community-wide engagement. During the quarantine, tele-health platform was promoted and yoga was introduced online to the community. Researches on yoga have indicated positive effects on medical and psychological complaints. While there are many physical activities that can be done at home, yoga was given the primary considerations, not only because it can be facilitated online but it is a well-researched craft with many existing literatures, and scriptures that supports its physical and mental health benefits. It is a practice that can be adopted by anyone anywhere while combating most of the modern day diseases that we face today, all at the same time.

References

[1] https://pubmed.ncbi.nlm.nih.gov/25030795/

[3] https://www.researchgate.net/publication/343139930

[4] https://www.researchgate.net/publication/350178349

[5] https://indjst.org/articles/evaluation-of-impact-of-ethics-of-yoga-in-the-psychological-health-of-college-students-a-randomized-control-trial

[6] Wiese, Christine et al. "Effects of Yoga Asana Practice Approach on Types of Benefits Experienced." International journal of yoga vol. 12,3 (2019): 218-225. doi:10.4103/ijoy.IJOY_81_18

[7] Sharma, Vivek Kumar et al. "Effect of fast and slow pranayama on perceived stress and cardiovascular parameters in young health-care students." International journal of yoga vol. 6,2 (2013): 104-10. doi:10.4103/0973-6131.113400

Chapter 3

Yoga & Your Body: How It Supports 11 Vital Organ Systems

Are you someone who likes to go on long drives? Isn't it fun to smoothly travel through beautiful terrain? How does it make you feel to drive or sit in a car that has sufficient fuel and reliable machinery? A healthy body allows you to move through life more efficiently. The human body has a complex machinery of its own. As you are aware, your body is more than just a mass; it is also responsible for allowing you to taste things, climb a mountain, and remember information. It is not only about what the human body is made up of, but also about its functions. Along with the cells, tissues, and organs that make up the whole structure of our bodies, we possess fully developed physiological systems that carry out several vital functions. As with cars, it is critical to maintain your body's engine by using the proper fuel, keeping it in operation to prevent rusting, and regularly checking for smooth operation. If you find something lacking, it only makes sense to get the right support or expertise.

The human body operates on various physiological systems. Now imagine a car factory for once. You're likely to witness various teams carrying out a variety of tasks. One group can be in charge of making the steering wheels, another might be making the seats, and a different team might be assembling the different parts of the engine. Similarly, as you might remember having studied in your secondary school, our body works on 11 organ systems, namely

The influence of yoga on the 11 organ systems is a fascinating interplay supported by numerous research studies. Here's a glimpse into how yoga affects these systems:

- Circulatory System: Research published in the European Journal of Preventive Cardiology (2015) suggests that yoga practices contribute to improved cardiovascular health, reducing the risk of heart disease.
- Respiratory System: Studies, including one from the Journal of Physical Therapy Science (2016), indicate that yoga enhances respiratory function, promoting better lung capacity and efficiency.
- Nervous System: The Journal of Clinical Psychology (2018) highlights yoga's impact on the nervous system, pointing to reduced stress levels and improved mental well-being.
- Digestive System: A study in the World Journal of Gastroenterology (2014) underscores how yoga aids in digestive health, alleviating issues such as irritable bowel syndrome (IBS).
- Muscular System: The Journal of Physical Activity and Health (2016) discusses the positive effects of yoga on muscle strength, flexibility, and overall musculoskeletal health.
- Endocrine System: Research in the International Journal of Yoga (2011) emphasizes the role of yoga in balancing hormonal activity, supporting the endocrine system's proper functioning.

- Excretory System: Evidence from the Journal of Renal Nutrition (2014) suggests that certain yoga postures may enhance kidney function and contribute to the overall health of the excretory system.
- Reproductive System: The Journal of Sex Medicine (2010) explores the benefits of yoga in addressing reproductive health concerns, including increased fertility and improved sexual well-being.
- Integumentary System (Skin): Dermatology Research and Practice (2016) discusses the potential of yoga to promote healthy skin through improved blood circulation and stress reduction.
- Immune System: The Journal of Behavioral Medicine (2018) notes that yoga's stress-relieving effects positively impact the immune system, enhancing overall immune function.
- Skeletal System: A study in Topics in Geriatric Rehabilitation (2016) indicates that yoga supports bone health, contributing to improved density and reducing the risk of osteoporosis.

These research findings collectively showcase how yoga serves as a holistic practice, benefiting not only physical health but also promoting mental and emotional well-being across all 11 organ systems

Like inside the car factory, different teams perform different tasks, but they all share a common goal: to make cars. So do the different systems within your body, responsible for different jobs, yet they all share the common goal of keeping you alive and let you experience the best of the world.

Our physiological system works for us every second of the day. If it stops working properly, we will have difficulty living our best lives. In other words, our body suffers from a blockage or a disease that limits its ability to effectively function. To reduce such discomfort, regular yoga practice has shown significant benefits in improving the regulation of the sympathetic and parasympathetic nervous systems. Modern-day research has shown positive shifts in the brain's composition, a stronger immune system, and healing effects on connective tissues through yoga. It can have a beneficial effect on each of our organ systems separately and holistically at the same time.

Cardiovascular system

If the bodily functions represent a factory, then the heart will lead as the foreman of the show. The heart lies at the centre of all the activities. The cardiovascular system consists of the heart and the blood vessel circulation system. "Circulation" is derived from the word "circular," which means "circle." Your body's heart, lungs, and blood vessels work together to form a closed loop through which blood flows. This system is responsible for three main functions, all of which are designed to keep your blood flowing throughout your body at all times. The pulmonary circulatory system governs your lungs; the coronary circulatory system governs your heart; and the systemic circulatory system governs the rest of your body. Each circulatory system, like the car factory teams, must accomplish its work independently in order for the circulatory system to function as a whole.

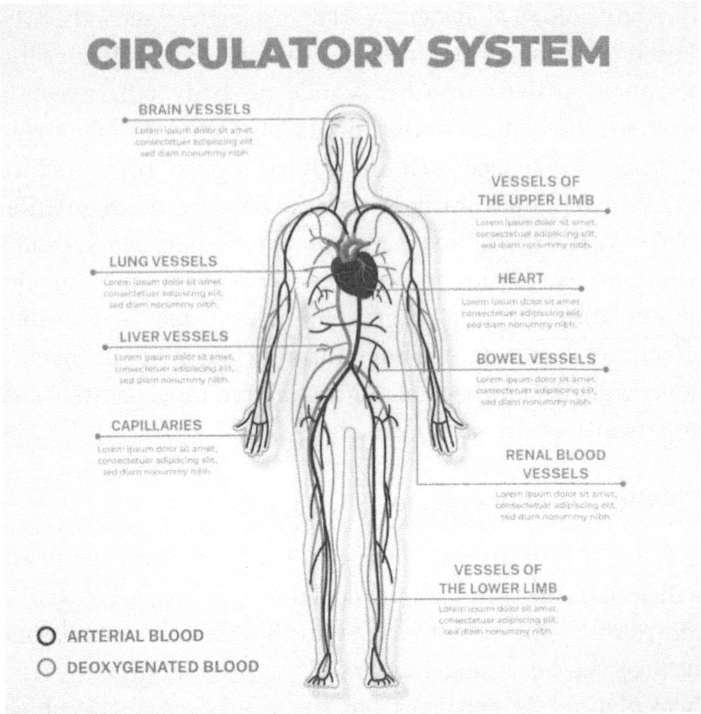

The problem arises when we start giving into toxic habits and unhealthy food diets, e.g. physical inactivity, harmful use of alcohol and tobacco, which show up as severe consequences such as blood pressure, raised blood glucose, raised blood lipids, and overweight and obesity. It can lead to diseases like coronary artery disease (CAD), which occurs when coronary arteries struggle to supply the heart with enough blood, oxygen, and nutrients. Cholesterol deposits or plaque build-ups narrow your arteries, decreasing blood flow to your heart. This can cause chest pain, shortness of breath, or even a heart attack.

It's true that physical activity revs up your heart, which can help manage or prevent heart diseases, but calming down the body and mind is important for the heart too.

"A large number of studies show that yoga benefits many aspects of cardiovascular health," says Hugh Calkins, M.D., director of the Cardiac Arrhythmia Service at Johns Hopkins [1]. "There's been a major shift in the last five years or so in the number of cardiologists and other professionals recognising that these benefits are real." One of the most significant causes of heart disease remains to be smoking. Some research shows that yoga could be an effective aid for smokers who want to quit. According to another study, slow-paced yoga session thrice a week reduced the incidence of cardiac arrhythmia episodes in patients with the illness. Another study found that patients with heart failure who participated in an eight-week yoga programme improved their exercise capacity and quality of life. They also had reduced levels of inflammatory markers in their blood, which relates to heart disease. Since stress is one of the leading causes of heart blockages, the breathing practises of yoga can help to relax the mind. There are some yoga poses that help to improve blood circulation in the heart area. Various specific asanas enhance the heart's functionality by supplying it with fresh oxygenated blood, like forward bend, bridge pose, and shoulder stand. These yoga poses aid in the removal of toxins from the body as well as the elimination of stress.

Some of the asanas for good heart health are:

1. Padangustasana
2. Uttanasana
3. Trikonasana

4. Veerbhadrasana
5. Bhujangasana
6. Setu bandhasana
7. Paschimosttasana

Pulmonary/Respiratory system

Did you know you can hear the pulmonary circulation? Yes, the vibrating beats you hear when using a stethoscope are the sound of the ventricles contracting and the heart valves shutting as part of the circulation process. The respiratory system includes the nasal cavity, pharynx, larynx, trachea, bronchi, bronchioles, and lungs (alveoli). Pulmonary circulation is the transfer of blood from the right side of the heart to the lungs and then back through the left side of the heart. Fresh, oxygen-rich blood enters the pulmonary veins before returning to the heart via the left atrium to re-enter the organ. The oxygen-rich blood then travels through a one-way valve into the left ventricle before exiting through the aorta, the heart's major artery. The left ventricle contracts, forcing blood into the aorta and allowing it to continue its journey throughout the body. It's worth noting that one-way valves are essential for stopping blood from flowing backward. The blood gases (oxygen and carbon dioxide) may mix if blood starts flowing in the wrong direction, posing a major hazard to your body.

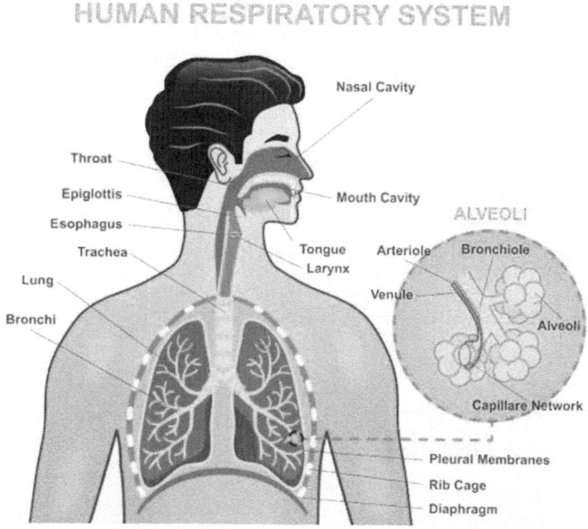

Yoga has a significant and positive impact on the respiratory system. Pranayama, or breathing techniques, has been found to enhance oxygen intake by up to five times. The more oxygen-rich blood that reaches the brain, heart, lungs, and digestive organs, the better these organs will perform and the better your health will be. Breathing exercises are not only beneficial to the respiratory system's function but they can also help with issues such as sinusitis, asthma, hay fever, shortness of breath, and allergies. Apart from breathing exercises, physical yoga poses help the respiratory system do its job by expanding the lungs and providing them space to breathe, engaging different body parts and boosting blood flow so that oxygen can reach the tips of your toes. Backbends and most standing postures in yoga open up the chest region, which not only relaxes the tightened muscles in that area but also allows one to use portions of the lungs that had previously been "occupied" due to bad posture, emotional tension, and environmental influences. Circulation throughout the body is significantly affected by inverted positions, and areas above the heart region receive an enhanced flow of blood as a result. Lastly, since all the body's systems are interconnected, focusing on yoga asanas that directly improve one system will have an impact on other physiological systems and the body as a whole.

Some of the asanas for good heart health are:

1. Bhujagasana
2. Usttrasana
3. Matsyasana
4. Trikonasana
5. Hasta uttanasana

Lymphatic system

If you have ever pricked a swollen blister on your foot during your childhood years, you have seen the lymphatic fluid. The lymphatic system produces a pale, slightly sticky liquid called lymph. The lymphatic system is an important element of the circulatory system that aids in the absorption of nutrients and the removal of waste. White blood cells make up the majority of lymph. Lymph is formed when blood plasma escapes from blood vessels and is absorbed into the surrounding tissue. Throughout the body, the fluid gathers in lymph tubes. The fluid is returned to the blood after passing through a lymph node to deposit trash. The waste deposits are collected in lymph nodes, which are clumps of tissue. A healthy lymphatic system is essential for a strong immune system. When not taken care of, your immune system can begin to respond erratically, much like a child in a candy store. This is when symptoms begin to emerge, including joint inflammation, allergies, cold extremities, depression, bloating, mental fog, and chronic fatigue. To make matters worse, a sluggish immune system can also contribute to weight gain. In case you didn't know, your lymphatic system and immune system are best friends. So if one isn't acting appropriately, chances are the other isn't either. Interruptions in the flow of lymphatic fluid can lead to very serious conditions like cancer, autoimmune disorders, and lymphedema.

Deep breathing exercises help you improve the flow of your lymph system, thereby helping the body get rid of toxins. Unlike the circulatory system, which is driven by the pump of the heart, the lymphatic system depends on gravity as well as on tissues contracting to squeeze fluid through its vessels. As a result, yoga poses like twists, forward folds, side bends, and inversions are ideal for increasing lymph flow [2].Yoga is particularly beneficial because of its ability to both target these congested lymph areas, managing the breath as a pump and also helping to regulate stress, which has been shown to decrease the immune response. Yoga incorporates the practise of gently compressing some of these lymphatic tissues to encourage lymphatic fluid circulation. The lymphatic flow of the extremities and torso, which works against gravity, is greatly aided by inversions. Because the diaphragm acts as a major pump for the lymphatic vessels, using diaphragmatic breath exercises and breath-centric movements while practising yoga helps to enhance the lymphatic benefits. A practise that involves inversion, squeezes, and stretches around the tissues surrounding lymph node clusters in the neck, armpits, and groin can greatly help in supporting a healthy lymphatic system and boosting your immunity. Numerous research studies that are being conducted on the effects of yoga on breast cancer patients have shown favourable results for small controlled groups [3].

Some of the asanas for Lymphatic health are:

1. Adho mukhashavsana
2. Anjayenasana
3. Dhanurasana
4. Sarvangasana
5. Leg up the wall
6. Veerbadhrasana 3

Muscular system

Do you think you can move every muscle in your body? The answer is, not voluntarily. There are some muscles that move involuntarily. The muscular system consists of three muscle types; smooth, cardiac, and skeletal muscles. Smooth muscle can be found in blood vessel walls and hollow organs like the stomach or intestines. The heart muscle, or myocardium, is made up of cardiac muscle cells. Skeletal muscles are connected to the body's bones. Only skeletal muscles can be controlled consciously and allow us to move our bodies, whereas the function of the other two muscle types is completely unconscious and governed by the autonomic nervous system. Skeletal and cardiac muscle fibres are grouped in a striped pattern, thus also called "striated muscle." Non-striated muscles are smooth muscles because they lack repetitive stripes.

MUSCULAR SYSTEM

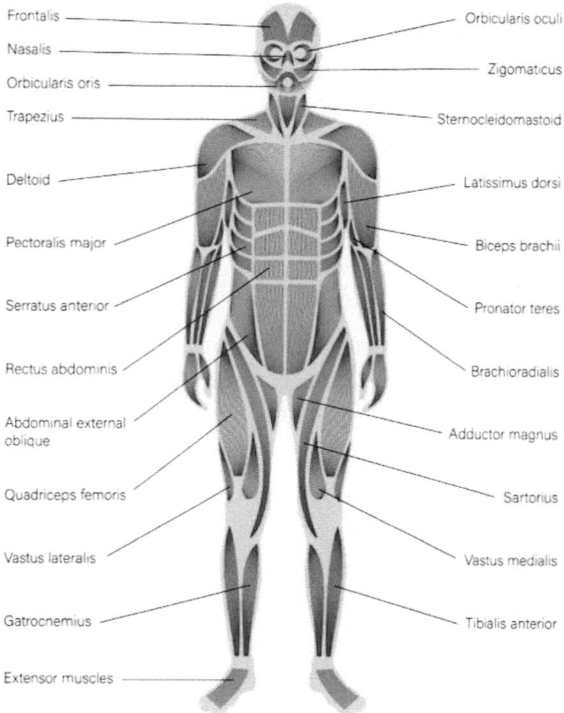

The human body is made up of an infinite number of cells that form tissues, organs, and systems. Yoga helps to keep the tissues around the joints in good shape. Similarly, it loosens the tissues and increases their flexibility. Yoga gives your body greater room. Furthermore, yoga helps to change the flow of the body, which helps to reduce stiffness. Water makes up 60% of our body weight. Our bodies' compressive forces are created by the fluid in our joints and spinal column, which provides shock absorption. More movement keeps the tissues hydrated, which keeps us from feeling stiff. Better flexibility means a wider range of motion, which minimises the chances of injuries and allows you to get the most out of your fitness regimen. Flexibility allows you to get the most out of your workouts. If your tendons and muscles are too tight, it could literally affect your skeletal structure. Consider people who spend their days hunched over a desk; their muscles become so accustomed to that hunched position that they lose the flexibility needed to allow the spine to sit up straight!

Consider a beaded bracelet on an elastic string: if you stick 20 cm beads onto a 15 cm elastic string, the beads will curve inward because the strand wouldn't be long enough to accommodate the complete length. The beads will sit in a beautiful straight line if you pull on both ends of the string until it reaches a length of 20 cm. This is how you position your bones in the ideal posture for your body by lengthening your muscle fibres. Numerous studies show how yoga plays an essential role in such bodily functions. A paper published in the journal of International Scientific Yoga on 'Yoga for Children with Disabilities' discussed how, through yoga, children can learn how to relax, focus their energy and develop poise, strength, balance and flexibility. They can learn how to develop mindfulness and self-awareness. Yoga practise can improve the mental and motor skills of children with learning and developmental disabilities. [4]

Some of the asanas for muscular health are:

1. Trikonasana
2. Dandasana

3. Navkasana
4. Ardha Pincha Mayurasana
5. Veer bhadrasana 2
6. Hastapadasana

Skeletal System

Like the aerodynamic structure of an aeroplane, the human body relies on a skeletal frame. This frame not only gives it a structure but also helps in the mechanism of all its functions. The human skeletal system is made up of bones and cartilage. The axial and appendicular bones make up the whole skeleton. The bones of the head and trunk form the axial skeleton. The limbs, as well as the supporting pectoral and pelvic girdles, make up the appendicular skeleton. An adult human body contains 206 bones. The joint, also known as the articulation, is the point where two bones come together. Cartilages support joints, which are reinforced by ligaments. Functions of the skeletal system include mechanical support, movement, protection, blood cell generation, calcium storage, and endocrine modulation. The skeletal system's components are adapted to the function of the bodily portion they support.

Human Skeletal System

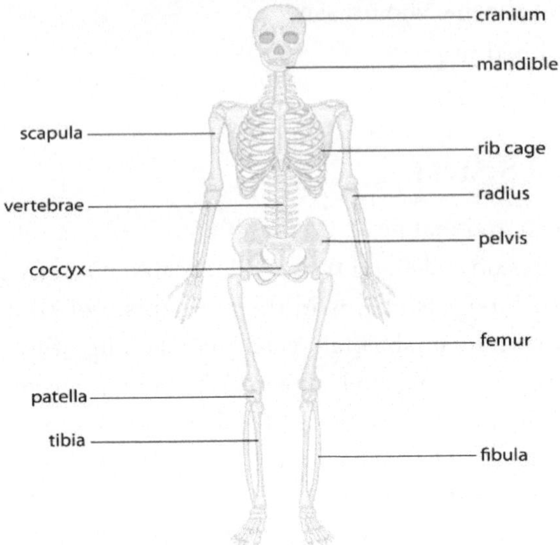

Yoga enhances the amount of lubricant in the joints, ligaments, and tendons. It is more reasonable to do yoga because it is low-impact as the asanas emphasise precision and proper alignment. Because the poses are held for a specific amount of time, the body has an opportunity to enhance blood flow and provide important supplies to all areas of the body. They also aid in the correcting and balancing of the functions played by the joints, ligaments, and tendons in giving the support that the body's limbs require to function properly. It's critical that your joints stay lubricated because if they don't, they'll start to limit your movement and make you more vulnerable to injury. Yoga's gentle pushes and controlled movements reach deep into aching joints. Furthermore, the controlled stretches, when combined with deep breathing exercises, relax and release the muscles that have tightened up around the joints in order to protect them. Studies have shown that a wide range of poses in the yogic system can be used to strengthen bones in various parts of the body. As a form of exercise to build strong bones, yoga is a complete workout and, as all the poses can be adapted and modified, there is no limitation to who can perform any of the poses and still get the required results while working at their own pace.

Some of the asanas for Skeletal health are:

1. Padangustasana
2. Dandasana
3. Kapotasana/ Rajkapotasana
4. Trikonasana
5. Hanumanasana
6. Malasana
7. Veerbhadrasana 1

Digestive system

We all know that during festival, weddings, parties and night-outs is the time when our digestive system goes through the most amount of pressure with all the kinds of food that we eat and beverages that we drink. The digestive system's job is to break down food into smaller and smaller components so that they can be absorbed and used as energy by the body. It is made up of organs from the gastrointestinal system as well as other digestive organs. The organs of the digestive system extend from the mouth to the anal canal. The mouth, pharynx, oesophagus, stomach, small intestine, large intestine, and anal canal are all connected by a tube. The tongue, salivary glands, pancreas, liver, and gallbladder are all accessory digestive organs that help in mechanical and chemical food digestion.

The ancient yogis recognised the importance of excellent digestion in maintaining radiant health and attempted to comprehend the mind-body link. Yoga can help us learn to breathe more deeply and relax our brains, which can contribute to better digestion. According to research most common psychosomatic symptoms of stress, nervousness, worry, and depression can even lead to digestive issues in many people. The digestive system is affected by a tumultuous mind. This is reflected in the effectiveness of our digestive system as a result. The food we eat has a significant impact on our ability to digest it. Yoga encourages the practitioner to become more aware of their surroundings. You gradually begin to choose meals that promote a sense of balance, harmony, and well-being—food that is natural and fresh, as well as wholegrains—rather than refined, fried, and processed foods. Overeating is a crime committed against the body, according to yogic science. As a result, it's best to eat slowly and deliberately. Dinner should be light and consumed at least 2 hours before bedtime. Continuous practise of yoga, including abdominal breathing and twists, can improve blood flow, prevent constipation and bloating, and help with the management of chronic conditions like irritable bowel syndrome (IBS) and gastroesophageal reflux disease (GRD). Such movements massage the internal organs of the digestive tract and strengthen the muscles around it.

INTERNAL HUMAN DIGESTIVE SYSTEM

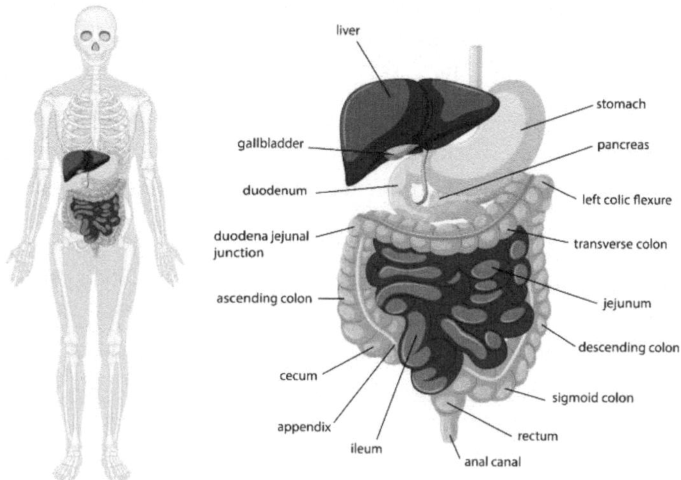

Some of the asanas for digestive health are:

1. Apanasana
2. Pawanmuktasana
3. Vajrasana
4. Triyak bhujagasana
5. Ardha Matsendrasana
6. Parivrtta Trikonasana

Nervous system

"Our nervous system helps us interact with the world. It includes the brain, spinal cord, and senses, all connected by tiny messengers called neurons. There are two main parts: the brain and spinal cord (central nervous system), and the nerves and synapses (peripheral nervous system).

The peripheral nervous system has two teams: the somatic nervous system (SNS) and the autonomic nervous system (ANS). The SNS lets us control our movements, like when you decide to kick a ball. It connects your body to the brain, sending messages about touch and movement. The ANS, on the other hand, works automatically, managing things inside your body, like your heart beat and stomach digesting food.

The ANS has two groups: the sympathetic (SANS) and parasympathetic (PANS). Imagine SANS as the "go, go, go" team during exciting moments, like playing sports. PANS is like the "rest and digest" team, taking charge when you relax or eat a meal."

"So, let's say you're playing your favourite game. When you need to run fast or make a quick move, your SANS kicks in, just like a superhero helping you react quickly. It's like the turbo boost for your body. But after the game, when you're chilling and enjoying a snack, that's when your PANS takes over. It's like the relaxation team, making sure your body calms down, and you can digest your food in peace.

HUMAN NERVOUS SYSTEM

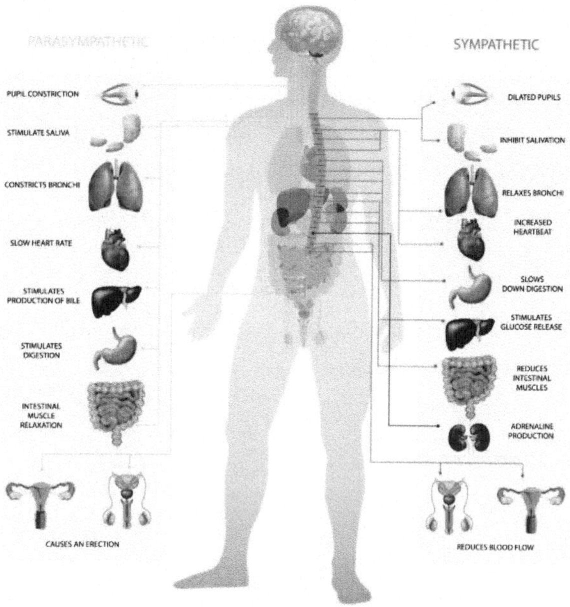

So, whether you're scoring goals on the field or chilling with friends, your nervous system is always there, making sure everything runs smoothly and keeping you in control – just like your own superhero team inside your body!"

A wrecked nervous system can act like fried wires, which can erupt into unpredictable responses at any moment when it is not necessary. Yoga can have both immediate and long-term effects on calming your nervous system. If you ask anyone who is an ardent meditator, he or she will tell you how meditative practises can help you soothe your mind within minutes, irrespective of how intense you might feel. Although it takes a bit of practise for sure, once you get the hang of it, it is only set to get better. It is safe to say that numerous research has been conducted which tells us about the great benefits of meditation and similar other practises within the yogic system that can help you calm your nervous system. All the 8 limbs of yoga allow nerve transmission from the body to the brain, which relieves mental and muscular tension. Including breathing exercises in your yoga workout routine can immensely aid in balancing the entire nervous system and support sufficient functioning.

Some of the asanas for Nerves system health are:

1. Balasana
2. Supta Badhakon asana
3. Supta Natrajasana
4. Vipreet karni
5. Ananda balasana
6. Setu bandhasana
7. Makrasana

Endocrine system

Think of the endocrine system as the body's own chemistry lab crew, carefully concocting the right mix of hormones for your well-being. This team, comprised of special organs called endocrine glands, operates like skilled chemists, ensuring the perfect blend of hormone flows throughout our body. These hormones act like chemical messengers, directing various essential activities.

Consider triiodothyronine as the lab's master recipe for regulating your body's metabolic system, like the chef ensuring the right cooking temperature. Meanwhile, estrogen and progesterone play the role of lab assistants, fine-tuning the chemical balance to regulate the menstrual cycle in women.

To send their chemical creations to different parts of the body, your hormonal lab crew releases these messengers directly into the bloodstream, much like carefully measured ingredients mixed in a flask. The team includes vital lab apparatuses such as the adrenal cortex, pituitary gland, hypothalamus, pancreas, thyroid gland, parathyroid glands, and the testes or ovaries.

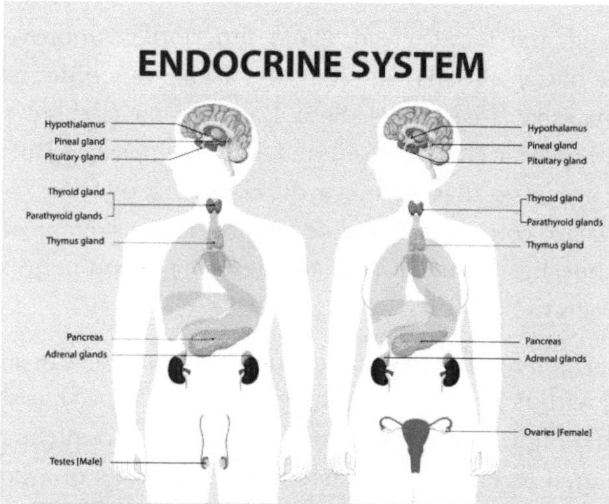

The endocrine system regulates various bodily functions through the secretion of hormones, which are chemical messengers that travel through the bloodstream to target organs. These hormones control processes such as growth, metabolism, reproduction, and stress responses, maintaining overall homeostasis.

Hormones act like chemical instructions traveling through the circulatory system, influencing crucial processes like growth, maintaining the right body temperature, and retaining hydration, much like carefully following a lab protocol. Occasionally, the hormonal lab encounters issues, like a test tube that doesn't react as expected.

Problems such as hormonal imbalance, thyroid irregularities, stress hormone surges (cortisol), insulin challenges, or early menopause are like experiments that need adjustment. But with the right care, your body's hormonal lab can tweak the formulas, ensuring a balanced and healthy outcome.

Such as standing forward bends, such as Sirsasana, increase blood flow to the brain, which improves the functioning of the brain and hypothalamus, as well as the pituitary and pineal glands.

Thyroid and parathyroid gland function is improved by poses like Halasana and Sarvangasana (shoulder stand) Matsyasana (Fish pose). Setu Bandhasana (Bridge pose), Bhujangasana (Cobra pose) and Badhakonasana (Butterfly pose) are poses that stimulate the testes and ovaries. Specific glands are compressed and decompressed in yoga postures, and this slight compression and decompression helps regulate secretions.

Modern research regarding endocrine parameters in adolescents with Polycystic Ovarian Syndrome (PCOS) has shown results highlighting improved menstrual frequency and hormonal levels with consistent interventions of a holistic yoga routine [5]. Scientific research conducted on cortisol levels during yoga Asanas has shown clear indications of Alpha wave activation resulting in a decreased amount of cortisol generation [6].

Some of the asanas for endocrine system

1. Bhujagasana
2. Ustrasana
3. Prasarita padottanasana
4. Malasana
5. Simhasana
6. Sarvangasana

Urinary/Excretory system

The excretory system can literally be called the poison-fighting team of your body. Believe it or not, your body contains poison. Untreated bodily waste can make you very sick. To guarantee that waste is taken away, your lungs, kidneys, and skin have to work together. Blood flows via the kidneys during systemic circulation. This part of the systemic circulatory system is also called the renal circulation. The kidneys filter a large amount of waste from the blood during this period. Your kidneys produce approximately 1.5 litres of waste every day, which is excreted as urine. Blood transports waste gases like carbon dioxide to the lungs, where they are exhaled and the body is also cleansed of waste from dead cells and sweat.

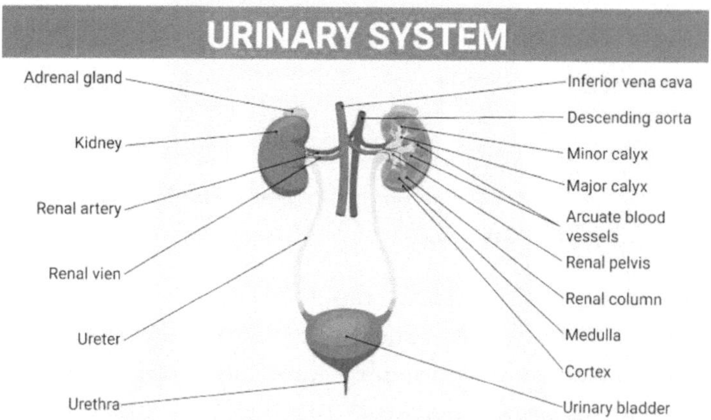

The kidneys play a critical function in the removal of poisons from our bodies. Any disruption in the creation, collection, storage, or expulsion of urine from the body can cause the kidneys to become slow, or perhaps stop working altogether. The ability to cleanse and maintain the health of our kidneys is critical to our overall health. Many urogenital system illnesses have been shown to be systematically relieved and overcome with the correct application of specific yoga practices and dietary adjustments. Research has shown that yoga improves sympathetic nerve activity, which reduces blood pressure. This in turn improves the excretory mechanism and results in normalisation of water and electrolyte balance. Yoga programmes have been considered to have a safe and effective measure as an alternate therapy to conventional treatment modalities for improving renal function and sometimes even decreasing the need for dialysis.

Some of the asanas for urinary/Excretory system are:

1. Mandukasana
2. Tadasana
3. Triyak Bhujagasana
4. Triyak Tadasana
5. Malasana
6. Gomukhasana

Reproductive systems

One of the most complexly designed organ systems is the reproductive system. The reproductive system, often known as the genital system, is a collection of internal and external sex organs that work together to facilitate reproduction. The male reproductive system and the female reproductive system function differently.

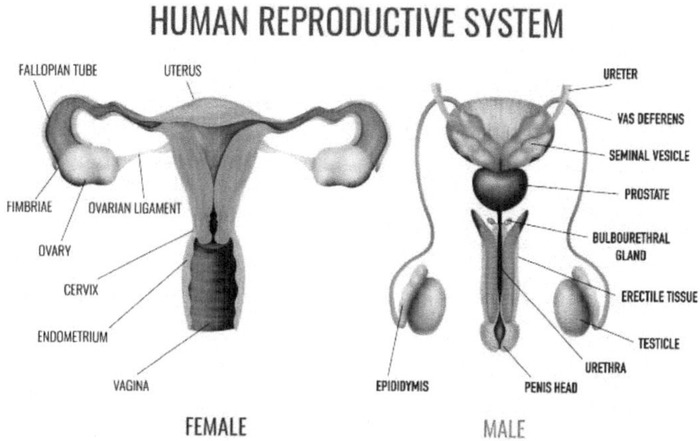

In women, the vagina is like a pathway that connects the outside of the body to the neck of the uterus (cervix). Inside, the ovaries produce hormones and eggs. These eggs travel to the uterus through the fallopian tubes. The uterus is like a special place that keeps and takes care of a developing baby. When it's time for the baby to be born, the uterus's muscles help push the baby out.

For men, there are external parts like the testes and penis. Inside, there's the epididymis, vas deferens (sperm duct), and some accessory glands. These parts do different jobs. The testes make sperm, the epididymis keeps them safe, and the vas deferens and other glands create a fluid that helps the sperm move. The penis, urethra, and vas deferens(Sperm duct) are all used for mating and putting the sperm in the right place.

According to research, wellness activities like yoga are beneficial in assisting couples navigate the ups and downs of the fertility journey. Yoga is an excellent way to assist your fertility, whether you are a seasoned yogi or a beginner. Combining fertility wellness treatments such as Yoga and Ayurveda has, cutting-edge infertility treatments that has proved to work wonders for many people. As you might know by now, yoga is reported to reduce stress and anxiety. Studies show that major changes to our lifestyles, diets, and activity levels over recent decades have impacted negatively on spermatogenesis in adulthood.

Sitting too much and being overweight can affect on your fertility.

Reduced Blood Flow: Prolonged sitting can decrease blood circulation to the pelvic region, potentially impairing the function of reproductive organs. Poor blood flow may disrupt hormonal balance, which is essential for fertility. Hormonal Imbalances: Excess weight often leads to hormonal changes, such as elevated estrogen levels in women or reduced testosterone levels in men. These imbalances can interfere with ovulation in women and sperm production in men.

Increased Risk of Chronic Conditions: Being overweight increases the likelihood of developing conditions like polycystic ovary syndrome (PCOS) in women or erectile dysfunction in men. Both can significantly hinder fertility.

Impact on Sperm Health: For men, sitting for long periods, especially with heat exposure (e.g., in tight clothing or on heated seats), can negatively affect sperm quality and motility, reducing the chances of conception.

Inflammation and Insulin Resistance: Obesity and sedentary lifestyles are associated with inflammation and insulin resistance, both of which can impair reproductive health and the ability to conceive.

Stress and Mental Health: A sedentary lifestyle combined with weight gain may lead to increased stress and anxiety, which can also affect fertility.

- Yoga is like a science which helps your body work better.

  Yoga is science that not only helps your body relax but also makes reproductive system work better. Starting yoga early is like giving your body a head start. Yoga is like a superhero for both men and women. In simple terms, sitting too much, being overweight, pollution and adult ratio in food can make it hard for your bodies to function properly. But doing yoga is like power back-up that keeps everything working smoothly.

Some of the asanas for Reproductive system are:

1. Badhakonasana
2. Paschimottasana
3. Sarvangasana
4. Halasana
5. Dhanurasna

Integumentary system

The skin not only protects the body but also serves another important purpose. It also removes dead cells and perspiration, both of which include waste materials. The excretory system relies on the integumentary system to remove waste via the skin. Dead epidermal cells accumulate in hair, fingernails, and toenails. These are evacuated through the integumentary system. Hair and nails grow as more cells die and are eliminated.

INTEGUMENTARY SYSTEM

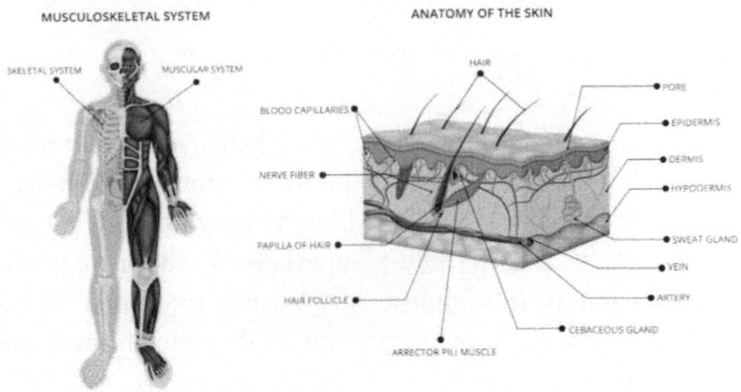

The skin is the body's biggest organ. The epidermis, dermis, and hypodermis are the three layers that make up the skin. They are like three sheets of cloth spread one over another. The first one is the epidermis. It is a multicellular epithelium that is thickly keratinised. The dermis is the second layer, which acts as a layer of connective tissue like glue beneath the epidermis, containing blood vessels and nerves that nourish the skin. The hypodermis is the third layer of skin consisting of fat, connective tissue, and skin appendages that make up the underlying fascia (hair, nails, sebaceous, and sweat glands).

Your skin has an important part to play in the improvement of your skin. Your skin, and particularly your face, suffers from a stressful lifestyle just like the rest of your body. Expect hormonal swings in the form of breakouts and other skin issues. If you don't eat properly or indulge in a hectic lifestyle. The science of yoga, on the other hand, has a huge impact on both the body and the psyche, which also results in healthy skin. Regular practise of yoga can help rid the skin of toxins and preventing carcinogenic chemical absorption and irregular hormonal outbursts.

Yoga also provides benefits through its more receptive and restorative styles. It supports the physiological systems of the body in a myriad of ways. Several yoga poses can be practised together to create a routine that specifically targets a particular organ system. It repairs and rejuvenate its functioning. That being said, one cannot simply attend one yoga class and expect to see cellular changes in their body. To fix all kinds of imbalances in our bodies, we need to practise yoga regularly over a period of time.

Some Asanas for the Integumentary system are:

1. Simhasana
2. Utthita Parsvakonasana
3. Shashankasana
4. Chakrasana
5. Kapol shakti vikasak
6. Shalbhasan

Chapter 4
The Pineal Gland Mystery: Unlocking Your Inner Light

Pineal Gland's Location: The pineal gland is a small part deep inside our brain. It's in the middle, where the two halves of the brain meet. The gland itself is quite small, measuring about a third of an inch in length and located at the centre of the brain. It is reddish-grey in colour and is primarily made up of pineal cells and neuroglia cells. The pineal gland has a lot of calcium, which makes it show up clearly in pictures taken by special machines (like X-rays). Doctors use this glands picture to find the middle part of the brain in these pictures, kind of like a helpful marker.

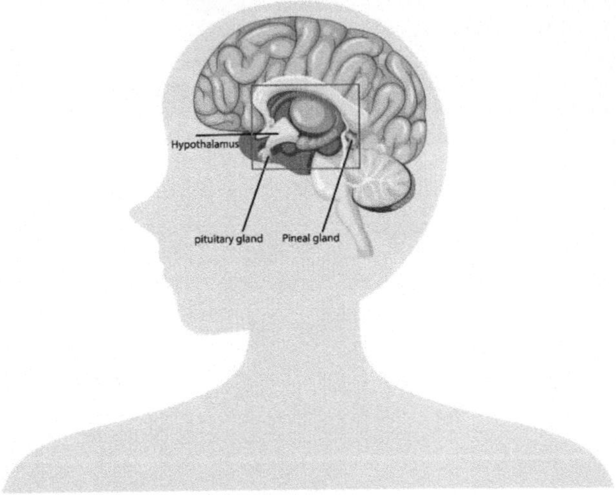

According to the research

Cerebrospinal fluid surrounds the pineal gland. Fluoride from water or pesticides accumulates at a higher rate in the pineal gland than in any other part of the body. Excess fluoride and other mineral deposits frequently cause pineal gland calcification or hardening. As a result, the body's ability to regulate melatonin as well as its circadian rhythm may be compromised. Due to the photosensitivity of the pineal gland, it secretes less melatonin during the day and more at night, which explains why most people are awake during the day and sleepy at night.

Scientists are also curious about what else this little gland does. Some studies suggest it might be linked to how we feel. For example, it could be connected to why some people feel a bit down during certain times of the year, like winter.

If not anything else, one thing has become increasingly clear to the modern psychologists and neuroscientists as they try to develop better tools to study the human brain, that there is far more to learn about the human mind than they currently know. In fact, scientists are still trying to find out more about the pineal gland today and experts have yet to determine its whole significance and function. This gland is found in nearly every species, and its function has long been unknown. The function of this tiny gland was one of the last to be discovered, and it is only now beginning to be understood.

Pineal Gland and Yoga

In simple terms, the pineal gland is like a puzzle for scientists today. They're still figuring out how it works and what it does. But interestingly, in Hinduism, they've got a clear idea about it.

Imagine the pineal gland as a tiny dot in your brain. Scientists are not very clear about its functioning. They are trying to understand it because it's so small and mysterious.

Now, in Hinduism, They see the pineal gland as this special point in your brain, like a key to unlock something amazing which can help you create health and wealth. Health by healing and wealth by novel ideas and imaginations. They call it the "third eye" too. So, while scientists are still figuring out the mystery of the pineal gland, They are telling you the way to tap into the potential of the pineal gland through things like meditation and yoga, making it a bridge between your regular self and something more spiritual and advanced.

They've already got the knowledge and telling the pineal gland's potential. So, here you are - caught between the modern scientific quest and the ancient insights of yoga and meditation.

On the other hand, in Yoga, they view the pineal gland not just as a brain part but as a doorway to more profound knowledge. It's a bit like having an ancient treasure map that guides you on how to navigate this small but mighty organ in your brain.

In Yoga (Asana, Pranayama, Kriya, Dhyana, Japa and more) help you connect with your pineal gland. It's not just about understanding it; it's about using it to tap into a deeper level of awareness and spirituality.

At this point, generations of Indian yogis and Rishis have firmly stood their position, on how yoga helps an individual to remove blockages from the chakra system and provides a therapeutic effect to the mind and body. Meditation is a popular method for stimulating the pineal gland and awakening the third eye. Meditation is said to activate the parasympathetic nervous system. It relaxes the body and mind so that daily worries do not interfere with living a happy and healthy life.

According to one study, people who meditate have higher levels of melatonin than people who do not meditate. Closing one's eyes during meditation increases the brain's perception of darkness, which could explain why this occurs.

The activation of the third eye chakra gives us a better understanding of the effects of yoga on the pineal gland. Alpha wave emissions are said to make the mind calmer and more focused. Other effects of such activation include a significantly improved attention span, as well as a dramatic improvement in focus and attention to detail. People have also reported that their senses sharpen, allowing them to be more aware of their surroundings.

The senses of sight, hearing, and taste have all been seen to improve. Ajna (Third eye chakra) chakra activation might initially generate impatience and rage. However, this is similar to cleaning a chimney, where all the accumulated filth has to be removed at once. Once these pass, you'll notice that you're at ease, and rage doesn't bother you as much as it used to. Consistent third eye activation results in a deep sensation of calmness in the mind. One of the most common signs of third eye activation is a sense of devotion.

Origin of Meditation

The Vigyan Bhairav Tantra is an ancient spiritual text that is part of the Shaivite tradition, associated with Lord Shiva. The name can be translated as "The Science of Divine Awareness" or "The Technique of Transcendental Knowledge." VIGYANA BHAIRAVA TANTRA means the technique of going beyond. VIGYANA means consciousness, BHAIRAVA means a state beyond consciousness, and TANTRA means the method: a way to go beyond consciousness.

It is essentially a manual on meditation and self-realisation, offering 112 techniques or methods to transcend ordinary consciousness and reach a state of divine awareness.

The text is a conversation between Lord Shiva and his consort, Devi Parvati (referred to as Bhairavi). In this dialogue, Parvati seeks guidance on understanding the nature of reality, consciousness, and the path to enlightenment. Shiva responds by sharing various meditation techniques that are simple, practical, and universal in nature.

Key Features of the Vigyan Bhairav Tantra:

1. Non-Dual Philosophy: The text emphasises the unity of the individual soul (Atman) with the universal consciousness (Brahman).

2. Practical Techniques: The 112 methods range from focusing on breath, sound, and sensory experiences to more abstract practices like contemplation of emptiness or awareness of the present moment.

3. Universality: These methods do not require specific rituals or adherence to a particular religion; they are designed to be accessible to anyone seeking spiritual growth.

4. Focus on Direct Experience: The Tantra stresses experiencing reality directly rather than relying on intellectual knowledge or dogmatic beliefs.

Which method will work for you?

Just know that generally, only 2–3 techniques will resonate with your soul and understanding! So, have patience and wait for the right technique!

Love and surrender are the most crucial elements for achieving the goal of these techniques.

Today, let me guide you on the first technique - 'After breath comes in – that is, down – and just before turning out – that is, going up – THB BENEFICENCE.'

Understand that your entire system operates through breath! Inhale consciously and exhale consciously. Observe your breath carefully - both incoming and outgoing breaths. Now, breathe in completely, and before the breath goes out, observe that there is a gap between the two. Just before the breath turns outward, there is a moment with no state of mind, no body mind – a sudden stoppage. You are not breathing (just holding the breath), and the gap between the two is very brief, but you need to be attentive. Be with that gap. When you are in that gap, no thoughts will flow, and nothing will appear in front of you because you are in no-breath mode - no mind mode.

Essence of wisdom - The whole universe can be experienced in the gap between breathing in and out."

Though there are numerous meditation styles, "Mindfulness Meditation," "Transcendental Meditation," and "Kundalini Meditation" are among the most well-known in the West.

All these meditations are in 112 meditative technique given Vigyan Bhairav Tantra. As part of traditional culture, more than 60% of the Indian population practises some form of meditation, either directly or indirectly. Yoga and meditation are taught in most schools throughout India. For example, in India, the Vethathiri Maharishi Institute for Spiritual and Institutional Education (VISION) has developed a comprehensive Yoga curriculum that begins in kindergarten and ends with a Ph.D.

The Indian government has created a Ministry with a budget solely dedicated to Yoga and Ayurvedic research. The benefits of yoga have recently gained widespread acceptance in the Western world. Harvard, MIT, and Yale have all encouraged research into this new medium. The NIH has set aside funds for this study as part of the National Centre for Complementary and Alternative Medicine (NCCAM). Many of these meditation techniques are employed for various purposes, and studies have revealed that they have varied neurophysiological effects. Because meditation is most commonly used to relieve tension and anxiety. It is typically regarded as a sort of relaxation treatment rather than a substitute for standard drug-based medicine.

References

- Fenton, Crystal. The Healing Power of the Pineal Gland: Exercises and Meditations to Detoxify, Decalcify, and Activate Your Third Eye. Simon and Schuster, 2022.

- https://www.deccanherald.com/content/573768/yoga-pineal-gland.html

- https://www.spiritualresearchfoundation.org/spiritual-research/

Chapter 5
Building Your Yoga Routine: A Step-by-Step Guide

Now that you understand how Yoga can reform your life, let's talk about starting out, especially if you're new to it. It can feel a bit confusing and tricky at first, not knowing where to dive in. Your current life might be a world away from what you dream of, or maybe you're kind of in the middle. You might have given it a shot before but didn't quite get there. It doesn't matter where you're starting from; what counts is that spark to begin. So, whether you're taking the first step or peeking into the world of yoga, what truly matters is the eagerness to kick off the journey. Get ready for a yoga adventure – it's not about where you begin; it's about embracing the excitement of starting the journey

Yoga is not exclusive; it does not matter how old you are, how much you weigh, what you do for a career, where you reside, or what religion you practice to be able to practice yoga. Yoga is suitable for almost everyone. Practicing yoga on a daily basis is a commitment to yourself and your personal development. Daily practice is necessary to maintain your physical fitness, mental balance, spiritual connection, and emotional strength. It's an easy-to-do, minimal and cost-effective practice that can be performed practically at any place. It doesn't have to be hard or time-consuming. Although ideally it is recommended to devote at least 50 minutes to yoga daily even if you take out 20 minutes per day, it will help your body, mind, and spirit.

Now that you have reached this stage of transforming yourself into a yoga Sadhak or Sadhika, it is my duty to hold your hand through the process of becoming one. The only way to incorporate yoga into your everyday routine is to make it a habit in order to reap its juiciest fruits. The key to building any habit for that matter, has to do with focusing on developing a new identity. Simply said, your current identity is reflected in your current activities. What you do right now is a reflection of the kind of person you think you are. The identity you hold right now already aligns with becoming a better human being. As a reader of this book, it is enough evidence that you have devoted as much time and energy to learn more about something that will help you improve your health and lifestyle. To fully and effortlessly make a new positive change, you need to get rid of the old negative thought patterns and behaviours. Once you overcome any of the limiting beliefs hindering you from building new habits. You can easily slide yourself into a more desirable lifestyle of your own choice.

Making A Change in Identity

Changing who you are starts with changing what you do. Often, we kick off this process by setting goals like "I want to lose weight" or "I want to build more muscle." Goals are like the finish line – they're what you get after following certain steps. But here's the thing: the journey, the process, is about the actions you take to reach that finish line. Now, your identity is like the set of beliefs that guide how you want to live your life. Goals usually focus on the outcome, not on who you are.

So, many folks start changing habits by concentrating on what they want to achieve – the results. But this often tackles the surface-level habits, the things we do. It takes a lot of motivation to stick with these changes, especially when the rewards aren't immediate. In reality, most people find it tough to keep up with regular changes when the payoff isn't right around the corner.

So, instead of just fixating on goals, let's talk about identity. It's like the core of who you are, the beliefs that shape your life. When we solely focus on results, it's like trying to change the surface without diving into the deeper currents.

Now, making changes based on goals requires a ton of motivation. Imagine trying to hit the gym every day just to shed a few pounds or gain some muscle. It sounds good initially, but without instant rewards, most people find it hard to keep up the momentum.

But here's the secret sauce – if you shift your focus to your identity, to the kind of person you want to be, the game changes. Instead of saying, "I want to lose weight," you start thinking, "I am someone who values a healthy lifestyle." This shift makes the habits stickier because they're no longer just about hitting a target; they're about being true to who you are.

Sure, it might not give you instant gratification, but it lays the foundation for lasting change. It's like building a strong house – you invest time and effort, but once it's set, it's solid. Shifting your identity isn't an overnight gig, but it's a game-changer in making habits your lifestyle.

For example, you might be a person who suffers from stress, negative thoughts and anxiety. Often such a situation can feel very limiting, and you might assume that it is a part of your identity. Being in such a situation might feel helpless. In this case, your inner monologue will be "I am a negative person", or "I am an anxious person". Thus, you believe that it is a part of your identity.

Creating identity-based behaviour is a better alternative and a simple solution. With this strategy, we begin by concentrating on the person we want to become. If you want to make a long-lasting change, there needs to be a shift on a deeper level. There are two ways you can make change in your behaviour.

One way is to start from the outer surface to the inner core, that is to set goals and try to achieve them, for e.g. You want to lose weight. Now, you follow a workout routine, a diet plan and take required supplements. Maybe you follow it for a week or over a few months. You might start to see some changes but then you get a big project at your job and you hardly get any time to devote to your health. Many people find it difficult to maintain such healthy habits for various reasons on a long-term basis. When you make a change right from the inner core towards the outer surface, it lasts longer, which means changing those limiting beliefs that are deep-seated within yourself. For e.g. when people say things like, "I am not a morning person", "I am not an athletic person", "I'm not good with numbers" or "I'm not a yoga person", they are limiting themselves by attaching those beliefs with their identity. This has to do with the kind of story they tell themselves regularly.

Nobody is born with such limiting beliefs, everyone learns and unlearns what they believed throughout their lives. This affects the identity one forms of them-self. If you do something every day, for e.g. You write daily, so you can say that you are a writer which is how it affects the kind of story you tell yourself. Once you have embodied an identity, the more you will repeat the actions required to maintain it, the more proof you will have to assure yourself of how you identify yourself, the more you will tell yourself the story about it. For e.g. "I am a writer, I write" or "I am a runner, I run". As soon as you start affirming, "I am a healthy person, I do yoga", the shift will start to take place right from that moment onwards. Here, you tackle the issue from the roots instead of using any kind of medicinal spray from the surface above.

Identity is nothing but what your brain repeats about what you are. Getting your brain to repeat these affirmative thoughts is the way to start. However, don't expect your thought process and identity to change overnight.

Alright, so here's the deal – changing yourself happens bit by bit. Think of it like planting seeds. You don't just throw them all in the ground and expect a full garden the next day, right? Same with transforming who you are. Patience is your superpower here.

Start with one thought and one piece of who you are at a time. It's like building with LEGO – one block at a time. You'll notice changes in yourself slowly but surely. First, one part of you will change, then another, and another. It's like upgrading different sections of your life.

Don't stress thinking your whole personality will do a 180 degree shift all at once. Remember, you built your identity piece by piece since you were a kid. Changing it works the same way – step by step. The magic is in taking small, steady steps towards your goal.

Thought

Now, you have learned how to tackle limiting beliefs from their roots. The next step requires you to align your thoughts with the identity, in order to create a new habit. Every individual is unique and everyone comes from a different background. Everyone has their own set of individual struggles and limiting beliefs. It is you who has to identify, who do you want to become. And then adopt those thoughts that contradict your limiting beliefs. In order to align yourself with a new habit, it requires two main steps:

- Identify who do you want to become?
- Align your thoughts with it by taking a small step everyday.

Our thoughts shape who you are and who you end up becoming. Thoughts often have huge effects on how you feel about a situation and task. Have you ever noticed when you are having a bad day, and you have given up on feeling better? However, a simple shift in your thought process can change your whole outlook on your day. It is difficult to turn the flow of your thoughts in a completely different direction. It might even seem forced when you start trying to think something positive. However, the key is to recognise your negative thoughts, and not to fight with them. Just let them come, and gently let them go. Then replace them with affirmative thoughts that align with the identity you want for yourself.

If you want to become a marathon runner, you need to start affirming yourself that you are a runner, first. Let go of any thoughts and beliefs that might stop you from becoming a runner. Yes, it might sound like easier said than done but changing your beliefs at a mental level is not as hard as you might think. It is how the identity becomes aligned with thoughts. That is why it becomes easier for actions to follow through on their own. Similarly, in order to do yoga regularly, you can start adopting such thoughts and beliefs that strengthen your identity as a healthier person, for e.g. "I am a yoga person, I live a healthy lifestyle". See, it's not just words; it's a mantra, a pledge to your evolving identity.

For any person with a nine to five job, it might seem extremely difficult to start taking some time out for a yoga session, early in the morning. You might be going to bed late at night after catching up on your favourite Netflix shows, Amazon prime series or watching reels. If you are also someone who frequently gives into their midnight cravings. Then waking up half asleep or partially groggy in the mornings. And then preparing for a morning yoga session might seem like climbing an Everest, at first. But you should not worry, this has happened to many people especially during the lockdown period. The wires of our body clocks have gotten fried with the 'work from home' daily routine and online classes. Most of the time sitting in front of your laptops finishing up your work late at night. What is more important right now, is how does one make better lifestyle choices from now onwards. This is where the idea of adopting an identity becomes helpful. For e.g. some affirmations that can help a person start living a healthier lifestyle are, "I am healthy", "I am grateful for everything that I have", "I have an abundance of energy", "I am open to learn new things", "I trust myself", "I am peace and calm", "I am mindful of each breath".

You may wonder, what after this? You have adopted a new identity but how are you going to make sure that it is implemented? This is why, thought is the next most crucial step of the process. Since you are going to bring about a change from within, it is important that you start making conscious choices about the thoughts that you entertain in your mind. Mindfulness is the key to this step. Become mindfully aware of your thoughts and then you will start becoming mindful of your actions, automatically. A change that happens to begin from the inner core towards the outer surface helps realign your belief system. As you start to see yourself in a better light about the beliefs that you hold regarding your health, the sooner you will see changes happening within and around you. As you start making conscious choices and repeating affirmations, the more it will start taking space in your subconscious. This is how one step at a time works. The new mindset will make its way in your life. This is how you will establish your new habits for a healthier life.

You can also alter this step as per your specific condition, say you are a patient with thyroid. You might feel tired easily, gaining a lot of weight, feeling depressed and having severe muscle aches. These are all common symptoms for someone suffering from thyroid. To start making better choices, in order to cure yourself of this condition in the long term, one can begin to adopt affirmations in a step by step manner. Such as, you decide to lead a healthier lifestyle so you adopt affirmations like, "I am a healthy person" or "I live a healthy lifestyle". Next, you might want to start doing yoga every day and use affirmations like, "I am a yoga person" or "I do yoga every morning" or "Yoga heals me". You would also want to make sure that you are taking the right nutrition to keep your hormones in check and eat the right food that will help your condition, using affirmations like, "I don't eat milk based protein and eat fruits everyday" or "The nutrition I take cures me of my thyroid symptoms" or "I eat clean and healthy food" or "I have a healthy food habit". You might also want to start meditating to improve mindfulness and mental health by adopting affirmations such as, "I meditate daily" or "Meditating for ten minutes every day helps me improve my mental health". This is how you can begin tackling your limiting beliefs and start living a healthier life. This step helps you make conscious decisions in your everyday life to start living a healthier life.

Plan

After aligning your thoughts with your identity, a plan-of-action can help you stay focused. To build any habit you need a supportive environment that help you stay on track. Creating a plan for your day, week or month can help you build your habits slowly. These plans don't need to be very rigid either. Depending on your personality and way of doing things, your timetable can be as detailed or as simple as you want. For example, if you are someone who doesn't like to be bound by a minute-by-minute schedule, a simple to-do list for your day can help you achieving your goals. Or if you are someone who likes to plan each hour of your day, you can go about that way.

Let's say you want to become a yoga person and do yoga every day in the morning. It might feel like a daunting task to shift your schedule. when you have been in the habit of sleeping late and waking up late. Lot of people have a busy schedule where they struggle to make time for yoga. Your daily lives often leave you so tired that even giving attention to your health seems like an added task. After an entire day of work, Netflix often seems like a better idea than choosing yoga or meditation.

In such a scenario, it will be helpful if you include working on your health as an integral part of your day. It will help you a lot if you make a timetable and put it right beside your bed that says "do yoga at 6AM in the morning".And then putting an alarm. You can lay out your mat the night before and perhaps put your yoga outfit along with it that makes you feel comfortable and confident, to change into as soon as you wake up. You can also make external changes in the surroundings, for e.g. light a scented candle, put on a diffuser, and make a list of asanas that you will perform for your yoga routine. These do not have to be rituals but only supportive elements with the intention of making change towards a healthier lifestyle. Lastly, you must try to be around people who encourage and uplift you. There are communities online and offline who can support you, encourage you when you are off track and help you get back.

Commitment

This is one of the most crucial stage while building a new habit. Commitment goes back to the first step of establishing an identity. When you commit to that identity, it is then the story that you used to tell yourself starts to change. You strengthen the identity connected to your beliefs, the more often you repeat it. The only way to stick to those beliefs is by committing to it. And repeating them regularly in all the ways possible. Commitment helps you gather proof for your new identity.

Often procrastination can become a hurdle between you and your ideal lifestyle. In the grind of our daily lives, it's always easier to choose to scroll through social media or binge on Netflix rather than making healthy choices. You are guilty of giving in to procrastinating and letting go of your commitments. One can use various techniques to stay committed to habits, techniques such as:

5 Seconds Rule – whenever you find yourself slacking or thinking about skipping your yoga routine or for that matter any new habit you are trying to build, use this method. Catch yourself right there and count from 5 to 1, backward in such a manner 5-4-3-2-1., it's like you're gearing up for a launch, As soon as the counting stops, make it a point that you get on with your work allocated. This helps you give that last push you need to get it started. This push is just enough to overcome the last-minute mindset of giving into comfort rather than change.

You often find yourselves in situations where you need just a little push towards your goals. For example, when you are trying to wake up in the morning to practice yoga, it will be tempting to not leave the comfort of your blanket. The motivation that you need to get up from your bed might feel huge. This is where the 5 seconds rule will come to your rescue and give you that nudge to get out of your bed.

As you start counting backward from 5 to 1, it's creating a sense of urgency. You're literally counting down to action, and by the time you hit 1, it's a commitment – a promise to yourself that you'll get started. It's a psychological reset. Shifting your mindset from hesitation to determination.

The power lies in its simplicity. Instead of overthinking or letting procrastination take over, the countdown provides a quick, decisive moment. It's like saying, "Enough thinking, it's time to do." The moment you stop counting, there's this subtle but effective push to initiate the task you were contemplating.

It's exceptionally useful because it interrupts the cycle of negative thoughts and delays. You're creating a small window where hesitation doesn't get a chance to settle in. This method is about building momentum, taking that crucial first step, and often, that's the hardest part.

So, consider the countdown as your mental launchpad. It's a strategy to break through that initial resistance. Its a transition from thinking about doing something to actually doing it. It's your tool to make that last push, converting intentions into actions and embracing positive change!

Reward Yourself – If you observe closely, you will realise that almost every action that you take is tied to an outcome. For example, you work to get your salary, or you get into your car to get to your destination. Thus, in your brain activity is linked with reward. Therefore, to train your brain to stick to your schedule, you can make a system of rewarding yourself.

It's a way of training your brain to associate sticking to your schedule with something positive. It's like saying, "Hey, I did my yoga today, so I get some points!" It turns your routine into a game where you collect points for each win, making it a fun and motivating way to stay on track.

So, if you're trying to make a new habit stick, consider introducing habit points. It's a simple, effective strategy to give yourself a little pat on the back and create a positive connection between your actions and rewards.

For e.g. 5 habit points can mean letting yourself go for a spa day, for 10 habit points means go to meet your friends or talk to them over phone. You can also use material rewards instead of points, that can lead to instant gratification which is like buying new clothes after consistently doing yoga for a month.

You could also make a system of depriving yourself of these rewards or benefits when you fail to achieve your goal. For example, if you fail to do your morning yoga, you will stop yourself from hanging out with your friends, or you would not have your cheat meal. This way these fun activities become a reward after your Yoga session. Another way to go about this is to add an activity of similar measure in place of yoga. For example, if you miss your yoga session, you could take a 45-minute walk instead. This will stop you from completely slacking off your goal.

Small and Slow Steps are Better than Quitting-

Sometimes, trying to change a lot of things at once can be overwhelming, and it's something we all experience in one way or another. The trick is to begin with small, gradual steps.

For instance, let's say you're used to waking up late and not doing any exercise. If you suddenly decide to practice yoga every single day right from the start, it might set you up for frustration and disappointment. Instead, it's better to start with small, slow steps.

Take it easy and begin with something manageable, like two yoga sessions a week. This way, you give yourself room to adjust to the new schedule without feeling too overwhelmed. It's like taking a gentle approach, allowing you to ease into the changes smoothly.

By starting small, you're creating a more realistic and achievable goal. It's a way of setting yourself up for success by building a routine that you can sustain over time. So, remember, small steps can lead to big changes, and it's all about making progress at a pace that works for you.

Sometimes, despite putting in a lot of effort, life can get busy or motivation might take a dip. You might have successfully made yoga a daily routine, but then, due to a hectic work schedule or simply feeling unmotivated, you miss a day or two. Suddenly, getting back on track seems like a daunting task.

Here's the key: don't demand perfection from yourself. You don't always have to be in a rush; it's okay to take it slow when life gets overwhelming. Even if you miss a few days or temporarily stop, it's completely fine. What matters most is not giving up because of a setback.

Think of it like a journey. If you take a little detour, that doesn't mean you've failed. Just start again from where you left off. It's about progress, not perfection. Life is full of ups and downs, and it's okay to adjust your pace accordingly. The important thing is to keep going, even if you hit a speed bump. Remember, one setback doesn't define your entire journey. So, be kind to yourself and keep moving forward.

Now, as you follow these steps and align your thoughts with action, it will turn into your reality. As your new identity starts to take shape, it's like witnessing the unfolding of a version of yourself. That is ready to embrace new possibilities. This emerging identity is not just a concept; it's a tangible reality that is there to guide you toward potentials you might not have believed were achievable before.

Action

As you see, establishing an identity is a way to establish new habits, just as much new habits are a way of establishing a new identity. The process functions both ways, keeping this in mind the most practical way to change who you are is by changing what you do. Taking a plan-of-action only pushes you more towards the identity that you wish to create. When you take action in alignment with your identity and thoughts with planning and commitment, it is bound to make changes in your life. Nothing can stop a change produced in such a way, not even yourself. Some people might even be shocked as to how this can show results without caring about the outcomes.

For e.g. You want to run a marathon. You wish to create an identity of a runner in order to establish a new habit of running. You affirm yourself that, “I am a runner, I am going to run a marathon.” You repeatedly tell yourself the same story. This is when you take action and start running. It is only easier when you take it step by step. Now, as you start to repeat those actions regularly it becomes a part of your own identity.

Through this step, people can begin to see change happening in reality. when trying to incorporate healthy practices in their everyday lives. Once you have gone through all the previous stages and reach the ‘action stage’ it becomes much easier to see yourself in your new identity. If you are someone who has a corporate job and an extremely busy life, the inner work that goes into changing your identity and adopting new habits could seem a daunting task. Although, taking time out for yourself becomes all the more important, in this case. This is why starting from within, step by step can help you achieve desired change in your life.

Imagine someone saying, "I want to do yoga every day, but waking up early is tough with my job." It's a common situation when people try to adopt new habits by focusing only on the surface, like setting an action plan.

The problem arises when you skip the earlier steps – the inner work – and directly jump into action. It often leads to struggles like low motivation, disappointment, and feeling discouraged. However, when you take the time to address your inner thoughts and beliefs, step by step, necessary for adopting a new identity, the change happens more naturally.

In simpler terms, if you just try to change what you do without understanding and changing what you think and believe, it can be tough. But when you work on the inside, tackling your doubts and beliefs, adopting a new habit becomes smoother and more successful. It's like building a strong foundation before constructing a building – it ensures a more stable and lasting result.

A great way to make sure you keep doing these actions regularly is by joining a class or a studio. Whether it's a physical class or an online one, joining a class can be super helpful. You not only get to learn from experts but also increase your chances of sticking to it in the long run.

When you invest your time and money in something, it makes you more committed. For instance, sticking to a solo yoga schedule might be a bit challenging. However, if you join an online yoga class, it feels like you're in it together with others. This sense of community can keep you motivated.

Having 2-3 yoga classes per week becomes more doable and realistic when you're part of a class. It starts to become a regular part of your routine, almost like a habit you've learned. And here's the cool part – you might even start missing it if you skip a session. It becomes a natural and enjoyable part of your daily practice.

Let's say, this person with a hectic corporate job wants to make time for yoga everyday in the morning, Or a mother of 2 kids wants to do yoga for her PCOS/PCOD, Or a senior citizens with multiple health issues makes the decision to adopt the new identity of a healthier self. They start using affirmations to incorporate healthy practices in his life, such as "I am a healthy person", "I do yoga every day", "I take out at least an hour a day from my busy schedule to devote time to myself", "I sleep on time to get eight hours of sleep every night", "I eat healthy food" etc. They goes on to plan for accommodating these changes. Perhaps, they buys a yoga mat and some comfortable clothing to do yoga in. They might ask there friends to help them eat healthily and provide assistance if necessary. Then, they goes onto commit to their beliefs even more by joining a yoga class whether in a yoga studio nearby or even online.

Post-Covid-19 there are several online classes which are guided by professionals. These classes were especially affective during COVID-19 surges. There are several benefits of opting for an online Yoga class for a busy working professional:

- It saves efforts as you don't have to especially dress up and go out for a yoga session. You can practice yoga from the comfort of your home.
- It also saves time as you don't have to travel to a yoga studio. You could almost save an hour of traveling

back and forth, giving you more time for your busy schedule.

- You would also save money, as online classes are generally less expensive. You could also save on the traveling cost.
- It would help you follow the law of making it easy. Whenever you are trying to incorporate a new habit in your life, keeping it simple and easy would help you start. Since online classes require less effort, it will help you get you into a routine smoothly.

Instead of just watching YouTube videos, opting for online courses with a professional instructor is a smarter choice. Why? Because watching videos online doesn't ensure you're doing the exercises and asanas (Postures) correctly or maintaining the right form. In an online classes, you get guided and corrected by an instructor. They offer expert guidance on your alignment, correct your form, and even guide you on breathing techniques and muscle engagement. These technical details are hard to grasp on your own just from a YouTube video.

Another bonus is that the instructor keeps you accountable, helping you stick to your routine. When you follow all these steps, you naturally feel compelled to take actions that align with your identity of becoming a healthier person. This gradual approach, makes it easier to incorporate new changes into your life.

Thus making the journey more enjoyable and sustainable.

Lifestyle

Once, the identity has been fully established and the action has been taken, you reach the last and final stage. Here you can find yourself having unlocked the potential, you had set to achieve in the first place. You make mindful choices as per the identity you have created for yourself. A healthy person would wake up early to do yoga everyday in the morning, start eating the right food, keep his or her surroundings clean. Although, a change in lifestyle is a process that happens gradually and takes time. But only when you are prepared to change.

Lifestyle is nothing but a consistent resolution. You need to be consistently resolving the issues that come up. You could make a blueprint for yourself about handling a problem based on the patterns. This would make the process of resolving the issues efficient. I have a formula that you can apply to multiple problems and find a solution to achieve a healthy lifestyle-

Healthy Lifestyle = Delight – Deficient

Let's unpack this formula and understand what this formula means. In this formula, delight stands for all the activities and habits that you enjoy irrespective of whether they are healthy or unhealthy. Consider "delight" as your positive assets. These are the activities that genuinely make you happy, boost your well-being, and contribute positively to your overall satisfaction. It could be anything from engaging in a hobby you love, spending quality time with loved ones, or practicing a form of exercise that brings you joy. These activities act as deposits in your well-being bank account, continuously adding to your positive balance.

These activities provide you enjoyment, and you love them. your subconscious mind has a natural preference for them and it gravitate towards them. For example, it could be getting a nice 8 hours of sleep, having delicious food, or enjoying your favourite TV show, etc

Deficient stands for all the activities that harm you and don't add anything to your goal of achieving a healthy lifestyle. These could be habits that compromise your health, hinder personal growth, or lead to unproductive outcomes. Such activities act as withdrawals from your well-being bank account, reducing your overall positive balance. These activities, though enjoyable, have a bad effect in the long run. They usually just provide momentary satisfaction and joy, but in reality decrease your delight in the longer period of time. For example, it may include waking up late, eating junk food, smoking, regular drinking or binge-watching shows while ignoring other responsibilities.

A healthy lifestyle is what you get when you subtract the 'Deficient' activities from the 'Delight' activities. This means you need to filter out all the activities that you enjoy that don't add anything towards your goal of being healthy. The goal is to maintain a positive balance by ensuring that your delightful activities outweigh the deficient ones. This involves making conscious choices to maximise the positive impact of your actions on your overall well-being. It's not about strict restrictions but about fostering a mindset that leans towards choices promoting long-term health and happiness.

Apply this formula to your daily decisions. Ask yourself whether a particular choice or activity contributes to your delight or falls into the deficient category. Gradually, strive to increase the delightful activities and decrease or eliminate the deficient ones.

By understanding and applying this formula, you gain a practical tool for cultivating a lifestyle centered around joy and health. It promotes a shift from short-term pleasure to long-term fulfillments, helping you make choices that align with your goal.

Now, let's understand this with the help of an example. Your 'Delight' activity is having delicious food. Everyone enjoys delicious food and having good food in itself doesn't stand in the way of a healthy lifestyle. But if you find junk food delicious and just want to consume that, then it would stop you from achieving your fitness goal. So, here the 'Deficient' activity is having junk food. So, according to the formula, if you minus junk food from your list of delicious food, it will help you achieve a healthy lifestyle.

Healthy Lifestyle = Good Food - Junk Food

Another example could be if your 'Delight' activity is getting proper sleep and feeling rested. In this case, the 'Deficient' activity standing in your way of achieving a healthy lifestyle with good sleep is going to sleep late. It would give you fewer hours of sleep and make you feel sleep deprived in the morning. Therefore, to achieve healthy lifestyle you need to subtract going to sleep late to achieve your healthy lifestyle with proper sleep and rest.

Healthy Lifestyle = Good Sleep - Going to Sleep Late

The key here is to identify the things that bring you joy and delight and the things that just provide you momentary joy but in reality, are deficient.

Another key point to keep in mind is the habit of 'Grab One, Throw One Out'. What this means is that you need to throw one thing out of your life to grab one thing into your life.

Even though this principle is seeing some popularity recently, it is not a new formula. It has been a part of our tradition since ancient times.

The 'Grab One, Throw One Out' principle is a powerful tool for crafting a healthier lifestyle. To better understand and apply this idea, let's break it down:

1. Tradition and Resolution:

This principle is not a new concept; it has roots in ancient traditions. Many cultural practices and religious rituals involve the idea of letting go of something undesirable to make room for positive changes. It has been a part of our tradition since ancient times. A lot of our religious and traditional practices are based on this principle. For example, elders used to take resolutions, while visiting a pilgrimage to leave one bad habit or practice when they wanted to manifest something in their lives. For instance, they would often take resolutions to abandon a bad habit or pattern when seeking positive transformations in their lives.

2. Application to Healthier Lifestyle:

To implement this principle for a healthier lifestyle, consider it as a method of creating space for good habits. It acknowledges the reality that you can't simply pile up new habits on top of existing ones. There needs to be a conscious effort to free up mental and physical space for positive changes.

3. Therapeutic Process:

The process of gradually letting go of one bad habit and replacing it with a good one can be therapeutic. It's a journey where you witness tangible changes step by step. This not only makes the transformation more manageable but also allows you to track and celebrate your progress. It's like de-cluttering your life – removing what no longer serves you to make room for what uplifts and enriches your well-being.

4. Practical Analogy:

The analogy of your life being like a computer or mobile phone storage reinforces the practicality of this principle. If you continuously add new apps without deleting old files, your system becomes sluggish and inefficient. Similarly, in life, if you keep accumulating habits without eliminating the counterproductive ones, it can lead to overwhelm and hinder your progress.

5. Balancing Act:

It's a delicate balance of recognising what habits are hindering your growth and being willing to release them to embrace healthier alternatives. The principle encourages a mindful and intentional approach to lifestyle changes, for sustainable and positive transformation.

In essence, 'Grab One, Throw One Out' is not just a rule; it's a philosophy that encourages a thoughtful and systematic approach to building a healthier, more fulfilling life. It's about making conscious choices, creating space for positive habits, and enjoying the therapeutic process of gradual, meaningful change.

The way to apply this principle to achieve a healthy lifestyle is to leave one bad habit when you want to start with a good habit in your life. It is not possible to just grabbing on to new habits, even if they are good, without first freeing up space for these habits to grow.

6. Progress Tracking:

As you consciously let go of a negative habit and introduce a positive one, you become a witness to your own progress. It's like watching a transformation unfold right in front of your eyes. This tangible tracking of changes can be incredibly motivating and fulfilling. You see yourself moving away from habits that might have been holding you back, step by step.

7. Incremental Success:

Small victories matter. By focusing on one habit at a time, you celebrate incremental successes. Each replaced habit is a triumph, creating a positive cycle of achievement and motivation. This approach ensures that the journey towards a healthier lifestyle is not overwhelming but, series of manageable and fulfilling steps.

8. Behavioural Change:

The process taps into the psychology of behavioural change. Breaking down the journey into smaller, achievable steps makes it easier for your mind to adapt. It's a proven approach in psychology that facilitates sustainable and long-lasting behavioural changes.

In summary, the therapeutic nature of this process lies in its ability to offer a structured and mindful approach to personal growth. It's not just about changing habits; it's about evolving into a better version of yourself, one step at a time. The progress becomes a story you're actively writing, and the therapeutic benefit is not just the destination but the journey itself.

Once you transform your habits from mere thoughts in your mind to actual experiences in your daily life, they become effortless. Achieving this requires a dedicated commitment, following the steps from establishing your identity to shaping your thoughts, creating a plan, making a commitment, taking action, and finally, embracing a healthy lifestyle.

Throughout this journey, it's important to acknowledge that nobody is perfect. Slip-ups happen, and that's okay. There's a saying, 'Don't miss the forest for a tree,' which fits perfectly here. Don't let minor setbacks overshadow the numerous benefits that come with regularly practicing yoga or any positive habit.

Building a new identity and incorporating new habits might come with occasional challenges, but it's crucial not to give up. When setbacks occur, view them as a small part of a bigger picture. Remember, what matters most is getting back on track. If you stumble into a pit, brush off your knees, stand up, and continue your journey. It's the resilience to keep going that truly counts in the end.

References

- https://www.apa.org/topics/behavioral-health/healthy-lifestyle-changes

https://jamesclear.com/identity-based-habits

Chapter-6
The 5-Day Lifestyle Reset: Renew, Recharsge, Rebalance

Why structured lifestyle reset program is required?

In your fast-paced, modern lifestyle, the constant hustle and bustle often leave you with little time for self-care. Living on autopilot, you navigate through your days without pausing to consider the impact on your well-being. This lack of mindfulness can lead to the accumulation of toxins in your bodies.

Unhealthy Eating Practices: The convenience of fast food and processed meals can contribute to poor dietary choices. When you are caught up in the demands of daily life, opting for quick but nutritionally deficient options becomes a common practice.

Stress: The pressures of work, deadlines, and various responsibilities can result in heightened stress levels. Chronic stress not only takes a toll on your mental health but can also manifest physically, affecting your bodies at a cellular level.

Lack of Proper Sleep: A hectic schedule may lead to irregular sleep patterns or insufficient rest. The body relies on sleep for crucial processes like repair and regeneration. Without proper sleep, these processes are disrupted, impacting overall health.

Laziness and Inactivity: In some cases, a sedentary lifestyle or the reluctance to engage in physical activity can contribute to the accumulation of toxins. Exercise plays a key role in promoting circulation and supporting the body's natural detoxification processes.

Addressing these challenges involves carving out intentional moments for self-reflection and self-care. It means making mindful choices about what you eat, finding strategies to manage stress, prioritising adequate sleep, and incorporating physical activity into your routines. Creating a balance in your modern lifestyle is essential to prevent the build-up of toxins and promote overall well-being.

In the wake of increasing awareness regarding lifestyle-related health issues, many individuals are proactively taking steps to improve their well-being. Here are some common practices you might be engaging in:

Healthy Beverage Choices: You may be incorporating beverages like kombuchas, Buttermilk (Chaas), Kanji, Solkadi (Kokam curry), Shatavari (Shatavari tea), Triphala, Ragi Ambil, Rice Ambil etc into your routine. These are fermented drinks and herbs known for its potential health benefits, including probiotics that support gut health.

Hydration and Nutrition: Ensuring you consume 3-4 litres of water a day with soaked dry fruits for nutrition in your diet suggests a commitment to hydration and nutrient-rich foods. Staying well-hydrated and incorporating antioxidants can have positive effects on overall health.

Intermittent Fasting: Exploring intermittent fasting at home indicates an interest in alternative eating patterns. Intermittent fasting has been associated with potential health benefits, including weight management and improved metabolic health.

Structured Lifestyle Reset Program: Choosing to participate in a structured lifestyle reset program led by professionals signifies a commitment to a more organized and guided approach towards improving your overall lifestyle. These programs often provide comprehensive support and guidance for holistic well-being.

Regardless of the specific methods you choose, the common thread is a heightened awareness and concern for your health. It's about making informed choices, being proactive in adopting healthy habits, and seeking guidance when needed. Whether through individual practices or structured programs, the goal remains the same – to enhance your overall well-being and prevent lifestyle-related health issues.

The 5-day Lifestyle Reset workshop is a tailored program aimed at cleansing both your body and mind. Here's a closer look at what it entails

This workshop is designed to address various aspects of your lifestyle, recognising the interconnectedness of physical and mental well-being. It's not just about temporary fixes but about fostering long-term positive changes.

Think of it as an internal cleanse. The program likely incorporates practices and strategies to detoxify your body, promoting the elimination of toxins accumulated through daily life and unhealthy habits.

The emphasis on both body and mind suggests a holistic approach. Mental well-being is often intertwined with physical health, and this reset acknowledges the importance of nurturing both aspects for overall vitality.

The goal is to leave you feeling rejuvenated at the end of the 5-day journey. This could involve revitalising practices such as mindful eating, relaxation techniques, or perhaps specific dietary adjustments to promote optimal health.

Acknowledging that true change takes time and dedication, the program encourages small, consistent steps. Each day contributes to the overall process, recognising that even the tiniest efforts matter in the grand scheme of building a healthier lifestyle.

Your commitment to this workshop reflects a dedication to your health. It's an investment in yourself, recognising that well-being is a journey that requires attention, intention, and time.

The effectiveness of the workshop may be enhanced by its ability to cater to individual needs. Whether through personalised guidance, support, or tailored activities, the program likely aims to make the experience meaningful and relevant to each participant.

While the 5-day duration is a specific timeframe, the intention is likely to instil habits and practices that participants can carry forward beyond the workshop. The focus is not just on immediate results but on fostering sustainable changes for lasting health.

In essence, the 5-day lifestyle reset is more than a short-term fix – it's a journey toward comprehensive health and rejuvenation. It recognises that health is a dynamic process and that every step taken towards a healthier lifestyle contributes to a positive and transformative experience.

Day 1- Gut Reset

You might have come across the term "gut health" and wondered about its significance. It's not just about digesting food; a healthy gut plays a crucial role in your overall well-being. Research suggests that a well-balanced microbiome in the stomach is not only essential for proper digestion but also influences your immune system and mental health.

Indeed, the gut is often referred to as the "second brain." This intriguing concept highlights the significant influence the gut has on your overall well-being, extending beyond its role in digestion. The gut-brain connection underscores that the health of your digestive system can impact mental and emotional states, further emphasising the importance of maintaining a healthy gut for overall health.

In other words, a healthy gut does more than just process food – it contributes to the strength of your immune system and has an impact on your mental well-being. It's a reminder that taking care of your gut goes beyond just ensuring effective digestion; it's a key factor in supporting your overall health.

A "gut reset" tries to enhance digestive health by maintaining the microbiome balance in the gut. Studies have shown that many other elements of health, including immunity and inflammation, are influenced by gut flora. Depending on the type of gut microorganisms a person possesses, this influence may be favourable or unfavourable.

The intricate relationship between your diet and gut health extends beyond mere digestion. The types of foods you consume play a significant role in shaping the diverse communities of microorganisms residing in your gut. Diets rich in fats or sugars create an environment which contributes to bacteria that thrive on these elements, while fiber-rich diets encourage the flourishing of different bacteria deeper in the gut.

Imagine your gut as an ecosystem, with various microbial residents competing for sustenance with each meal you consume. The choices on your plate become a form of ecological management, influencing the delicate balance of these microbial communities.

Moreover, this microbial landscape is not just a bystander in your digestive process; it actively communicates with your body. The health of these microbial communities is linked to various aspects of your well-being. A balanced and diverse gut microbiome is associated not only with efficient digestion but also with a robust immune system and even mental health.

So, each time you sit down to a meal, you're not only nourishing yourself but also fostering an environment in which specific bacteria thrive. The implications of this reach far beyond digestion – they extend to the intricate interplay between diet, gut health, and your overall health. By making conscious dietary choices, you become an active participant in cultivating a gut environment that supports your well-being on multiple fronts.

However, now a question arises: what do we mean by gut?

What is the Gut?

When we talk about the "Gut," we're referring to the entire Gastrointestinal System, a journey that begins in the mouth and concludes at the anus. Contrary to a common misconception that the gut is solely the intestines, in reality it encompasses the full digestive tract.

The idea of a gut reset is sometimes misunderstood. It's not just about addressing microorganisms in the lower intestines; it involves a holistic approach. To achieve a successful detoxification of the body, the entire gastrointestinal tract must be considered in the reset process. This includes the mouth, where digestion initiates, and the stomach, where crucial processes occur before reaching the intestines.

A thorough gut reset understands that the well-being of your entire digestive system is key to overall health. By expanding the focus beyond just the intestines and including the complete gastrointestinal tract—from mouth to anus—you ensure a more comprehensive and effective approach to detoxification. This holistic perspective acknowledges that each part of the digestive journey plays a role in promoting a healthier gut. So, when considering a gut reset, it's not just about isolated regions; it's about nurturing the entire digestive system for a robust and lasting impact on your well-being.

Why is Gut Reset Important?

Our daily consumption of chemically processed foods, like refined flour, refined fats, trans fats, and sugar, accumulates over time and disrupts the natural microorganisms in the gut. The gut plays a crucial role in immune health, acting as a barrier against viruses, fungi, and harmful bacteria.

Taking care of your gut is like giving it a superhero cape because it does more than just digest food.

However, continuous exposure to unhealthy foods can lead to a condition known as a "leaky gut," where the defence barrier becomes permeable, allowing pathogens to enter the bloodstream and cause illness.

Conditions like irritable bowel syndrome (IBS), inflammatory bowel disease (IBD), and celiac disease can increase the risk of leaky gut, making the body more susceptible to infections.

Researchers demonstrate- your gut is like a mini control centre for your emotions. It talks to your brain, telling it how to feel through a nerve called the vagus nerve. This communication is what scientists call the gut-brain axis. Picture tiny messengers (your gut bacteria) sending signals to your brain, affecting how you feel and even how you make decisions.

But, when you are stressed, it's like a wild party in your gut. The messengers get confused, and your gut-brain connection can get a bit wonky. This can impact not just your stomach but also how you think and feel.

So, by treating your gut well, you are not only being kind to your stomach but also nurturing your emotional superhero side. It's like giving your body a powerful duo – a strong gut and a happy brain!

Now, here's where it gets interesting – these superhero bacteria are sensitive to hormones, which means stress can throw them off balance. It's like a little turbulence in the gut-brain communication system. When you're stressed, it might affect these tiny superheroes, creating an imbalance that can impact both your gut and your judgment.

So, in the grand adventure of your body, taking care of your gut means keeping these tiny superheroes happy and ensuring they continue to be excellent pilots for your overall well-being.

Post COVID, taking care of your gut becomes significant. Turns out, a lot of issues might actually start from gut. Research has found that making short-term changes to what you eat can quickly change the bacteria in your gut. In a study from 2013, they saw that when people switched to a plant-based diet, the bacteria in their gut responded fast.

So, a gut reset could be like hitting the refresh button for your health, helping with various issues that might be linked to your gut. It's like giving your body a fresh start after going through a tough time.

Forget about juggling various green juices and kombuchas for a detox. I've got something simpler – a detox drink that cleanses your system and gives your gut a fresh start. It's an easy way to reset your gut.

The recipe for this magic drink

Ingredients

1/2 teaspoon dhania seeds (Coriander seeds)

1/2 teaspoon jeera seeds (cumin seeds)

1/2 teaspoon sauf (Fennel seeds)

1 litre water

Add all the ingredients in water and boil it for 5 minutes. Strain it in a flask. Have it like tea in a cup, not a glass. Make sure you don't reheat it and drink it. Keeping a flask will be helpful to drink during the day for 3 to 4 times.

This drink is like a reset button for your gut, helping you feel rejuvenated without the hassle of managing multiple drinks. Sip your way to a healthier gut!

Day 2- Body Reset

When I say Body Reset I mean working on the "Prana Shakti" of the body, because without the "prana" the body is dead.

Pranayama" doesn't have a direct English translation, and that's because it's rooted in Sanskrit. It's a blend of "Prana," meaning vital energy, and "Ayama," meaning to lengthen or work on.

In the yoga realm, "Prana" isn't just a casual breath; it's the internal energy that keeps our bodies alive. Prana is powerhouse that maintains health, vigour, and vitality, flowing through chakras and nadis, which are energy centres and channels in the body, respectively.

So, how exactly is prana and breath related? According to ancient yogic teachings, breath is the vehicle for prana. Every inhalation draws in fresh pranic energy, while every exhalation releases stagnant or depleted energy from the body. This intimate relationship between breath and prana forms the foundation of many spiritual practices and healing modalities.

According to yogic wisdom, when this vital energy (Prana) faces roadblocks due to issues in chakras or nadis, it can lead to illness. Now, here's where breathing steps in as the hero.

The regulation and maintenance of Prana are deeply intertwined with how we breathe.

So, Pranayama isn't just about inhaling and exhaling; it's about tapping into this powerful life force, ensuring it flows freely, and keeping the body in harmony. It's like tuning into the rhythm of your internal energy for a symphony of health and well-being.

Now, let's talk about another key player in the body reset game – Kumbhak, which is essentially the art of holding your breath. Picture this: when you're gearing up to push a heavy table, you instinctively take a deep breath and hold it. That act of holding your breath for added strength – that's Kumbhak.

It's like building up an internal force within us by holding our breath. Imagine collecting this force, and when the time is right, unleashing it for tasks that need a bit of muscle.

Here's the magic – when you incorporate Kumbhak into your pranayama practice, you're not just working on surface-level stuff. You're diving deep into your vital organs, the powerhouses that keep your body ticking. Unlike your regular gym exercises or weightlifting that focus on muscles, pranayama with Kumbhak works on your vital organs.

Sure, you might hold your breath during other activities, but it's not as systematic or targeted. Pranayama with Kumbhak brings a mindful approach, ensuring a powerful impact on those organs that often don't get much attention in your regular fitness routines. It's like giving your internal organs a strength training session – a boost they truly deserve for optimal health.

In Lifestyle reset program, you're not just sticking to simple deep breathing; you're delving into the wisdom of ancient yogis. They've handed down a treasure of rhythmic deep breathing techniques, each with its own special effects on your mind and body.

Now, here's the important bit – these techniques are powerful, and you should learn them from a qualified teacher or professional. They're like the secret sauces of yoga, and a guide can show you when to practice, how many times, and for how long. It's like having a yoga guru by your side.

What is Pranayama?

Before Maharishi Patanjali delves into the eight limbs of Yoga, he drops a hint about pranayama in the first chapter of the Yoga Sutras. It's like a sneak peek before the main show. He explaining how to cleanse the mind, emphasising the connection between pranayama and purifying the mind.

Now, when he officially introduces pranayama in the second chapter, he places it as the fourth step in the Ashtanga Yoga journey. In a nutshell, he lays down the rules and benefits of pranayama in a series of sutras from 2:49 to 2:53.

First off, Patanjali makes it clear – pranayama is a sitting game. You need to be in Asana (a comfortable seated posture) before diving into the world of controlled breath. It's like setting the stage for the breath-work to unfold.

The Hatha Yoga Pradipika, an ancient text on Hatha yoga, also spills the beans: "Proper pranayama can wipe out diseases, but watch out – improper practice can invite trouble." The lungs, heart, and nerves can become your strong allies with the right pranayama.

But the essence remains – pranayama is a crucial step in the yoga journey, not just for the body but primarily for the mind. It's like a key that unlocks the door to a purified and focused mind. And, as with all things in yoga, there's a method to the madness, a sequence to follow, and a wisdom to guide the practice. So, in the grand tapestry of yoga, pranayama has its own special place, inviting us to sit, breathe, and embark on a journey within.

Why is Body Reset/Pranayama Important?

Emma Ferris, a physiotherapist and breathing coach, says 80 percent of the world's population breathes wrong or has a breathing dysfunction [2]. To check if you are among the majority of the population, there is a simple technique that you can do even while reading this book. Put one of your hands on your stomach, and take a deep breath in. Now, you have to notice if your belly deflated or inflated as you inhaled. Did you pull your belly inside? If so, you are breathing wrong. Why? When you take a breath, the breath should go up to your stomach and your stomach should inflate.

Researches show that most people only breathe right for 4 hours a day, and while they are sleeping. But this could be increased with the help of pranayama. If you are not doing pranayama on a daily basis, you are supposedly breathing wrong. Body Reset teaches you the correct way of doing pranayama, thus, correcting and unblocking the flow of your "prana", i.e. the functions of your body.

Pranayama also boosts immunity. Pranayama practice provides more oxygen to the blood, reduces stress levels and fights anxiety - all of which boost the immune system.

Pranayama is not only beneficial for your physical health, but also for your mental health. Pranayama considerably lowers anxiety and depressive symptoms. These changes are linked to altered connection and activity in the parts of the brain, which is responsible for processing emotions, paying attention, and being conscious. It helps you destress all of the stress that the modern lifestyle often makes you accumulate. Stress and mental health itself are linked to physical ailments like thyroid and diabetes. When compared to how our lives have altered, regular pranayama practice might have an even greater positive impact on our health and wellness.

Body Reset entails using pranayama to control and unblock the flow of prana (Vital energy) in your body. It is advised that everyone should include 15 minutes of pranayama in their schedule.

The term 'nadi' means channels, like pathways for life energy, and 'shodhana' means purification. So, 'nadi shodhana' is a practice to cleanse these channels. There are 72,000 astral channels, with Ida, Pingla, and Sushumana being the main ones.

The goal is to purify these channels for smooth energy flow. Nadi shodhan pranayama helps remove blockages in these channels, ensuring energy can flow freely.

So, seek guidance in chapter 7. It's the key to unlocking the full potential of these ancient breathing techniques and ensuring a safe and beneficial practice. Let the journey into the world of pranayama begin with wisdom and guidance!

Day 3- Mind Reset

It's essential to recognise the signs of mental exhaustion and take steps to reset. One effective method is to schedule short breaks throughout the day. These breaks allow your mind to recharge, helping maintain focus and productivity. Additionally, incorporating activities like deep breathing or a brief walk can be beneficial. Finding a balance in your schedule and prioritising self-care is crucial. For avoiding negative effects of constant busyness. Remember, taking care of your mental well-being is an investment in healthier work-life balance.

The best strategy to increase productivity and safeguard your mental health at the same time is to create a timetable. Which enables you to work less but more effectively. You need a strategy for taking a break from work in between periods of deep effort.

There are various ways to achieve a mind reset. And different techniques work for different people. Some find solace in activities like meditation or deep breathing exercises, while others prefer engaging in hobbies, spending time in nature, or simply taking a short walk.

The key is to disconnect temporarily from work or any stressors and engage in activities that bring a sense of peace and relaxation. This break allows your mind to reset, preventing burnout and promoting overall well-being. Incorporating regular mind resets into your routine is a proactive measure to maintain mental health in our fast-paced and demanding world.

Mind reset is a way of letting go of this accumulated stress. But a question arises: what do we exactly mean by mind reset?

What is Meditation?

Mind reset targets on resetting your mind and brain with the help of practice like meditation. Everyone can benefit from the straightforward practice of meditation, which can lower stress, improve relaxation, and foster peace. The benefits of meditation can start to manifest right away as you practice. Learning how to do it is simple.

Often, due to a lot of thoughts, you are not able to get a clear understanding of your situations and decisions. For example, if you are working on a project, and a lot is already going on in your mind, you won't be able to get clear thoughts about the plan for your work. In such a scenario, meditation helps you think reasonably. It is the art of detachment from stress and at the same time attachment to the whole universe. Meditation helps you organise your thoughts, have a clear picture of your goal for further planning and execution. Furthermore, meditation fosters emotional well-being by increasing self-awareness. Which allows you to manage your emotions more effectively. Over time, these improvements can lead to a greater sense of inner peace and fulfilment. As you continue to meditate, you may also experience better physical health, such as improved sleep, lower blood pressure, and a stronger immune system. Ultimately, meditation is a powerful tool for personal growth, helping you to live a more balanced, purposeful, and harmonious life.

Why is it Important?

In today's world, most of you rely more on mental effort than physical labour. Work environments have shifted from physically demanding tasks to mentally intensive ones. These often involves long hours at desks, screens, or in meetings. This shift makes meditation incredibly important for maintaining balance and well-being. The ways in which humans eat, sleep, communicate, and survive have all been significantly altered by farming, industry, and technology.

Your brains are unable to adapt to your changing way of life. Evolutionary psychologists refer to this as a "psychological mismatch," when the brain and its functions are no longer well suited for the contemporary world. Your capacity to adapt is impacted by this misalignment. You are now anxious, unhappy, and stressed out most of the time.

Meditation helps in tackling this misalignment between your brains and your lives. Meditation allows you to slow down. It will help you increase your intuitive skills. Over practice of being present in your current environment, you will notice much more calmness in yourself. It would also lead you to a healthier lifestyle. Once you learn how to be mindful, you are mindful through every act of yours. It teaches you to choose what is right for you, over your mental conditioning.

For example, our eating habits are increasingly becoming unhealthier. People often eat sitting in front of either Netflix or the television. So, even an important task like giving nourishment to your body that keeps you alive is sidelined. When you are mindful, you know what you are eating. Therefore, you will not overeat, and give your body the food that nourishes.

Think about your mind like a newly captured animal, let's say a dog. Now when you fasten it to a post, the dog is not pleased. He pulls against the rope for days while screaming, stomping, and trampling. He finally comes to terms with the fact that there is nothing he can do and settles down. You can start feeding him and taking care of him safely at this point. Over time, you can educate your dog to perform a variety of chores and completely do away with the rope and post. You now possess a trained dog.

In this analogy, the wild dog represents your wildly active mind, the rope represents mindfulness, and the post represents our meditation object, our breathing. The result of this procedure is a well-trained, focused mind that can be applied to the extremely difficult task of cutting through the layers of delusion that conceal reality. The mind is calmed by meditation.

Meditation works on mental health issues as well. Psychotherapists have recently started using mindfulness meditation as a key component of their treatment plans for a variety of issues, such as depression, substance addiction, eating disorders, marital problems, anxiety disorders, and obsessive-compulsive disorder.

Impact of Mind on Physical Health

It is a lesser-known fact, but the health of your physical body is also connected to your mind. Scientists have found that meditation practices have a variety of positive effects on physical health. In addition to reducing stress, meditation can treat high blood pressure, lessen chronic pain, enhance sleep, and soothe digestive problems.

All diseases come from your thought. An underlying thyroid issue may become worse under stress. Consider the situation when hypothyroidism runs in your family. Your body releases the hormone cortisol when you are under stress. The thyroid may have to work harder to produce enough thyroid hormone as a result of excessive cortisol, which can disrupt thyroid hormone production.

Your future health may be significantly impacted by untreated previous trauma. According to Harvard Medical School studies, the emotional and physical responses it sets off can increase your risk for significant health disorders like heart attack, stroke, obesity, diabetes, and cancer.

Our body has a unique way of holding onto stress and trauma, and it often manifests in specific areas. Joints, chest, throat, and pelvic regions are common places where this stored trauma can create blockages. Research indicates that women, in particular, may store trauma in their pelvic region, potentially leading to conditions like PCOS/PCOD.

There are many meditation techniques around the world. All of them are very well listed and explained in the ancient text "Bhairav Tantra" which has 112 meditation techniques. There is not a single meditation technique that is not mentioned in Bhairav Tantra.

The simplest way to start as a beginner, Watch your breath. Your breath is always with you. Paying attention to it keeps you in the present moment. Helping you forget about past problems and future worries.

Here's how you can do it: Sit down in a comfortable position every day and turn your attention inward. Notice what happens with each breath you take in and each breath you let out. For example:

- Length of Breath: Pay attention to how long each breath lasts. Is it short or long?
- Sensation: Notice what you feel when you breathe in through your nose or mouth. Is the air warm or cool?

- Location: Be aware of where you feel your breath the most. Is it in your chest, your stomach, or maybe your nose?

Don't think too hard about these questions, and don't try to change your breathing pattern. Just relax and become aware of these small details that you usually miss during your busy day.

As you focus on your breath, let your mind settle. If you get distracted by thoughts or noises, gently bring your attention back to your breath. It's natural for your mind to wander, but with practice, it will become easier to stay focused.

Here's a simple example to illustrate this process:

Imagine you're sitting in a quiet room. You close your eyes and start to breathe in slowly through your nose. You notice that the air feels cool as it enters your nostrils. You count the seconds as you breathe in: one, two, three, four. Then you exhale slowly through your mouth, and you feel the warm air leaving your body. You count again: one, two, three, four. You feel the rise and fall of your chest or belly with each breath. You might notice your shoulders relaxing or your muscles unwinding.

As you continue to breathe, you might hear a noise outside or remember something you need to do later. When this happens, don't get frustrated. Simply acknowledge the distraction and gently guide your attention back to your breath. Feel the air moving in and out, and let everything else fade into the background.

Day 4- Viprit Aahar

You've probably seen folks at weddings and parties eat anything they want without giving it any thought. The following day, many people begin experiencing Stomach aches, Acidity, Vomiting, Headaches, Nausea, etc. In reality, individuals rarely consider what shouldn't be eaten with what is during parties.

Viruddha Ahara is a unique concept from Ayurveda. This concept talks about how foods interact with each other and how they're processed. Ayurveda says that certain diets and their combinations can mess up your body's tissue metabolism and stop tissues from forming properly. They call these combinations Viruddha Anna, or incompatible diets. Foods can become incompatible if they're mixed wrongly, processed incorrectly, eaten in the wrong amounts, or at the wrong times or seasons. That's Viruddha Ahara. There are numerous foods that are healthy in nature but if mixed with certain food becomes unhealthy. Ayurveda has a number of food-related rules.

It has been specified which foods should not be combined under the Viprit Aahar. For some people, considering the country, time, fire, nature, dosha, age etc., some food items prove to be harmful. Such foods are included in the viprit aahar.

What is Viprit Aahar?

Some food items are harmful by nature, while some food items are such that alone are very beneficial and health enhancers. However, when these substances are mixed with any other food instead of benefiting, they harm health.

These are called Viruddha Aahaar or Viprit Aahaar(Incompatible food). Consuming viprit aahar can lead to many different types of diseases. This is because these substances together contaminate the blood, increase the doshas and disrupt the expulsion of the faeces(Human waste) from the body. It is said in Ayurveda that continuous consumption of this type of anti-diet might slowly affect the body and contaminate your body.

Ayurveda gives a list of food items that should not be eaten together:

Have you ever wondered why some foods leave you feeling bloated, sluggish, and just plain uncomfortable? According to Ayurveda, the ancient Indian system of medicine, the answer lies in the concept of incompatible food combinations.

In Ayurveda, every food has a unique taste, energy, and effect on the body. When certain foods are combined in a way that is not harmonious, they can create toxins in the body and disrupt the delicate balance of our doshas, or energy types.

The examples of incompatible food combinations according to Ayurveda? Let's take a look:

Combination	Reason in Ayurveda	Effect on Body
Fruit with Dairy	Fruit is cooling and cleansing; dairy is warming and nourishing.	Causes fermentation in the stomach and creates toxins.

Meat with Dairy	Meat is heavy and hard to digest; dairy is also heavy and can create mucus.	Leads to digestive issues and disrupts dosha balance.
Honey with Hot Liquids	Honey is cooling; hot liquids are warming.	Turns honey toxic, creating "ama" (toxins) in the body.
Raw and Cooked Food Together	Raw food is light and easy to digest; cooked food is heavier and takes longer to digest.	Causes digestive issues and overworks the digestive system.
Fruits with Grains	Fruits are cleansing; grains are nourishing.	Causes fermentation in the stomach and disrupts dosha balance.
Hot and Cold Food Together	Hot food stimulates digestion; cold food slows it down.	Causes digestive issues and disrupts dosha balance.
Milk with Sour or Fermented Foods	Milk is heavy and nourishing; sour/fermented foods are light and cleansing.	Causes indigestion, creates toxins, and disrupts dosha balance.

Bananas with Milk	Bananas are heavy and create mucus; milk is also heavy and hard to digest.	Causes digestive issues and creates toxins.
Nightshade Vegetables with Dairy	Nightshade vegetables (e.g., tomatoes, eggplant) are heating; dairy is cooling.	Causes digestive issues and disrupts dosha balance.
Beans with Cheese	Beans are heavy and hard to digest; cheese is also heavy and creates mucus.	Causes digestive issues and creates toxins in the body.

This table highlights the Ayurveda principles and potential effects on digestion when certain foods are combined.

Incompatibility/antagonistic (Viruddha-Aahara)

1. Veerya Viruddha (Potency Incompatibility)
    - Example: Fish + Milk
2. Sanskar Viruddha (Processing Incompatibility)
    - Example: Heated Honey
3. Matra Viruddha (Dose Incompatibility)
    - Example: Honey + Cow's Ghee in equal proportion
4. Krama Viruddha (Order Incompatibility)
    - Example: Hot water after taking honey
5. Kala Viruddha (Time Incompatibility)

- Example: Pungent substances in summer, cold substances in winter

6. Samyoga Viruddha (Combination Incompatibility)
   - Example: Fruit salad or Milk + Banana
7. Parihar Viruddha (Contraindication Incompatibility)
   - Example: Cold water after hot tea or coffee

Here's a table summarizing a Few more examples of incompatible foods and combinations:

Category	Incompatible Foods/Combinations	Effects/Notes
Milk Incompatibilities	Kalothi, Vari, Wala, Matki, Jaggery, Curd, Tamarind, Jamun, sour foods	Should not be eaten with milk.
	Garlic, green vegetables, radish	Excessive consumption can cause skin diseases.
	Milk after green vegetables or spices	Should not be consumed together.
	Milk in khichdi	Avoid adding milk to khichdi.
Curd Incompatibilities	Hot foods (jackfruit, fennel, bananas, fish, meat, chicken)	Should not be consumed alongside curd.
	Chicken or deer meat	Should not be eaten with curd.

	Different animal meats	Avoid cooking or eating together.
Specific Food Combinations	Radish with urad dal	Should not be eaten together.
	Honey with ghee, lard, oil, water	Limit proportion when consumed together.
	Lotus seeds with honey	Should not be eaten together.
Severe Health Risks	Aquatic meat with honey, jaggery, milk, radish, rice, broken grains	Can lead to vision problems, tremors, hearing loss, slurred speech, mental illness, and death.
Cooking Methods	Spinach cooked in sesame oil	Can cause diarrhea.
	Betel leaf after jackfruit	Should not be consumed together.
	Reheating oil and food	Leads to oxidation, increasing oxidative stress and producing harmful free radicals.

This table provides a clear overview of incompatible foods, their combinations, and the potential effects according to Ayurvedic principles.

Why is it Important?

People who keep on consuming the above-mentioned diets, their stool, impurities and body juices, etc. get distorted. They can end up being a victim of these types of diseases due to inflammation at a molecular level.

- skin diseases
- food poisoning
- impotence
- belching
- large boils
- fistula
- Stomach diseases
- hemorrhoid
- leprosy
- Tuberculosis
- Cold
- IBS
- Fatty liver

These are just a few basic examples of incompatible food combinations according to Ayurveda. By avoiding these combinations and focusing on eating foods that are harmonious with your doshas, you can improve your digestion, boost your energy, and promote overall wellbeing.

So next time you sit down to a meal, remember to consider the Ayurvedic principles of food combining and choose foods that will nourish and support your body, not harm it.

Day 5- Immunity Boosting

The immune system defends the body against infection and disease; it battles anything from common illnesses like the flu and colds to catastrophic disorders like cancer.

Our immune systems are intricate and subject to a variety of influences. Vaccines increase resistance to particular diseases. You can also boost your immune system by eating healthily, exercising, staying at a healthy weight, getting enough sleep, quitting smoking, and abstaining from excessive alcohol consumption.

Researches that support the claim of enhancing immunity with Massage.

The foundations of good health include balanced eating, enough rest, and consistent Yoga practice. However, incorporating self-massage into your daily or weekly regimen can further enhance your resilience.

Massage promotes relaxation and improves circulation. Additionally, measurable changes occur in the body's immune and endocrine systems.

A 2019 study by The Massage Centre found that a single session of massage can significantly increase white blood cell production, which is crucial for the body's ability to fight infection.

Furthermore, a 2015 study published in the International Journal of Therapeutic Massage & Bodywork demonstrated that regular massage sessions over four weeks led to sustained increases in lymphocyte count and improved immune function.

Another study from 2018, featured in the Journal of Alternative and Complementary Medicine, highlighted that massage therapy can reduce cortisol levels, thereby decreasing stress and enhancing overall immune response.

Additionally, a 2020 study published in Frontiers in Psychology reported that massage therapy improved sleep quality among participants, which is another critical factor in maintaining a robust immune system.

Furthermore, massage therapy has been shown to improve flexibility and range of motion, as evidenced by a 2021 study in the Journal of Bodywork and Movement Therapies. This study highlighted that athletes and individuals engaging in regular physical activity experienced enhanced performance and reduced injury rates when incorporating massage into their routines.

By integrating massage therapy into your health regimen, you can not only boost your immune system but also improve mental health, cardiovascular function, pain management, flexibility, and overall quality of life.

This holistic approach to wellness underscores the importance of considering complementary therapies like massage to support and enhance traditional health practices.

Evidence supports that there is increasing white blood cell production, reduction of cortisol levels, and enhancing lymphocyte counts.

According to clinical studies, regular massage improves the immune system's capacity to attack specific cells. While reducing the number of T cells in the body, which helps the immune system as a whole. Increased circulation and lymphatic movement carry beneficial nutrients throughout your body and filter metabolic waste. Since the lymphatic system doesn't move on its own, massage plays a crucial role in that. Studies have shown that massage can boost lymphocyte levels. They are immune system support cells that assist the body fight off pathogens.

There is evidence that stress significantly suppresses the immune system. One of the finest methods for lowering stress is massage since it lowers the level of the stress hormone cortisol.

The National Centre for Biotechnology Information claims that the immune system is adversely affected by pain. Massage has a significant impact on reducing discomfort. It help your body more easily fend off an illness.

Not all of us can afford the luxury of consistent massage therapy appointments with a professional. Thankfully, self-massage techniques like Abhyanga, acupressure, and dry brushing can be equally beneficial. Practice one or all of these three simple methods to benefit your health and mind.

1. Abhyangam: Abhyanga, in simple terms, refers to the practice of applying oil to the skin followed by a massage in specific directions. This technique holds significant importance in Ayurveda for various purposes. It can be performed as a self-massage as part of one's daily morning routine, known as Dinacharya, or conducted by a trained Panchakarma professional to treat a wide range of diseases affecting different systems of the body.

Daily Practice (Dinacharya)

When performed daily as a self-massage, abhyanga helps maintain overall health and well-being. The routine application of oil followed by a massage can:

- Enhance Circulation: The massage stimulates blood flow, ensuring that oxygen and nutrients are delivered to all parts of the body.
- Promote Detoxification: By stimulating the lymphatic system, abhyanga helps in the removal of toxins from the body.
- Improve Skin Health: Regular oil application moisturises and nourishes the skin, improving its texture and appearance.
- Reduce Stress: The rhythmic motions of the massage calm the nervous system, reducing stress and promoting relaxation.
- Boost Immunity: Enhanced circulation and lymphatic drainage support the immune system.

Therapeutic Use (Panchakarma)

When performed by a trained Panchakarma professional, abhyanga is tailored to treat specific health conditions. Depending on the individual's Prakriti (constitution) and the nature of the ailment, the practitioner selects appropriate oils and techniques to:

- Balance Doshas: The massage can help balance the body's doshas (Vata, Pitta, and Kapha), which is essential for maintaining health and treating diseases.
- Support Dhatus: Abhyanga supports the health of the body's tissues (dhatus). There are seven dhatus in Ayurveda: plasma (rasa), blood (rakta), muscle (mamsa), fat (medas), bone (asthi), bone marrow (majja), and reproductive tissue (shukra). Each dhatu

plays a critical role in the body's functioning, and abhyanga helps ensure their proper nourishment and maintenance.

- Alleviate Specific Conditions: Different oils and massage techniques can be used to address specific health issues such as joint pain, muscle tension, digestive disorders, and nervous system problems.

Practical Benefits of Abhyanga

1. Enhanced Muscle Tone: Regular abhyanga can improve muscle tone and strength by stimulating the tissues and enhancing circulation.
2. Joint Health: The massage helps lubricate the joints, reducing stiffness and improving flexibility.
3. Better Sleep: Abhyanga promotes relaxation and can help improve sleep quality.
4. Mental Clarity: The practice has a calming effect on the mind, leading to improved mental clarity and focus.
5. Youthful Appearance: By keeping the skin well-moisturised and nourished, abhyanga can help maintain a youthful appearance and reduce the signs of aging.

Customisation Based on Prakriti

In Ayurveda, it is crucial to customise abhyanga based on an individual's Prakriti (constitution). Each person has a unique balance of Vata, Pitta, and Kapha doshas, and the massage should be tailored to support this balance. For example:

- Vata Constitution: Individuals with a Vata constitution benefit from warm, heavy oils like sesame or almond oil. The massage should be gentle and calming.
- Pitta Constitution: For Pitta individuals, cooling oils like coconut or sunflower oil are ideal. The massage should be moderate and soothing.
- Kapha Constitution: Those with a Kapha constitution benefit from lighter, warming oils like mustard or corn oil. The massage should be vigorous to stimulate circulation.

Abhyanga is a holistic Ayurvedic practice that offers numerous health benefits when incorporated into daily routines or used therapeutically. By understanding and applying the principles of abhyanga, individuals can enhance their physical, mental, and emotional well-being. This ancient practice not only supports the health of the body's tissue but also promotes overall harmony and balance within the body and mind.

Dosha-specific oils are used in the Ayurvedic massage method known as abhyanga. It promotes healthy blood flow, lymphatic drainage, cleansing, stress reduction, and restful sleep. Abhyanga is usually done with sesame oil because it's the only oil (apart from ghee) that's able to penetrate all the seven dhatus of the body. The seven dhatus are the seven tissues of the body: plasma (rasa), blood (rakta), muscle (mamsa), fat (medas), bone marrow (majja), nerve tissue (asthi), and reproductive tissue (shukra). This oil has the ability to move through all of these tissues all the way to our bones. Great oils for Abhyanga include almond, coconut, sesame, castor oil, and ghee. These can be used singly or in combination. It becomes an even more effective treatment if you add essential oils that strengthen the immune system.

Your creaky joints may finally find ease. Because abhyanga (specifically with sesame oil) has a way of penetrating all our seven dhatus, it can be incredibly nourishing to joints that need a bit more lubrication.

Use circular strokes on joints, the abdomen, the chest, and the face, and lengthy, repetitive strokes on long bones—always working your way toward the heart. Do not forget about your feet and head.

Take your time removing the oil from your skin. Resting for 5 to 15 minutes following will allow the oil to fully absorb.

Sit in a steam or sauna if you have access to one. A light, dry towel can then be used to gently buff away any remaining surface oil. Take a warm shower with light soap if you need to be less oily.

Abhyanga takes longer than dry brushing, but it's certainly worth giving it a try once or twice a week.

2. Dry Brushing: The first line of defence against sickness is your skin. It functions as a barrier, aids in detoxification, and produces Vitamin D, a crucial component of immunity. The skin can't function correctly if its integrity is damaged or if dead cells are clogging its surface. In Ayurvedic medicine, dry brushing is referred to as Garshana. It exfoliates the skin, aids in the discharge of impurities by promoting blood and lymph flow, and, like any massage, helps lower stress.

You'll need cotton or towel gloves for a softer exfoliation or a delicate, natural-bristled brush. To promote lymph drainage, keep moving up from the feet and hands and always in the direction of the heart. On the back and the long bones of the arms, legs, and body, use lengthy strokes. Apply circular motions to the belly, chest, and joints. Your skin should turn just a little pink; do not apply excessive pressure, and take care around sensitive regions.

Depending on your needs and the constraints of your schedule, a dry brushing session should last anywhere from 5 to 15 minutes. Make sure to do it before your morning shower so you can wash any toxins and loosen skin cells.

Dry brushing not only benefits the skin but also supports overall health by stimulating the lymphatic system. The lymphatic system is responsible for transporting lymph, a fluid containing white blood cells that help fight infections. By promoting lymph flow, dry brushing aids in the removal of toxins and enhances immune function.

In addition to its immune-boosting properties, dry brushing can improve circulation, giving the skin a healthier appearance and a natural glow. The increased blood flow can also help reduce the appearance of cellulite by breaking down fat deposits beneath the skin. Regular dry brushing can lead to smoother, firmer skin over time.

Moreover, the practice of dry brushing can have a calming effect on the mind. The rhythmic, repetitive motions can be meditative, helping to reduce stress and promote relaxation. This aspect of dry brushing aligns with Ayurvedic principles, which emphasise the connection between physical and mental well-being.

To maximise the benefits of dry brushing, it is important to maintain a consistent routine. Integrating this practice into your daily or weekly self-care regimen can lead to significant improvements in skin health and overall wellness. Remember to follow up with a moisturiser after your shower to keep your skin hydrated and supple.

In summary, dry brushing is a simple yet effective technique that supports the skin's health and enhances the body's immune system. By incorporating this practice into your routine, you can enjoy smoother skin, improved circulation, reduced stress, and a strengthened immune response.

Materials Needed

- Dry Brush: Choose a brush with natural bristles for effective exfoliation. The bristles should be firm yet gentle to avoid damaging the skin.
- Gloves: Alternatively, you can use cotton or silk gloves for a softer exfoliation experience.

The Dry Brushing Process

1. Begin with the Feet: Start at the soles of your feet, using gentle, upward strokes. Move slowly and methodically, covering each part of your foot before progressing to the next area.
2. Brush Towards the Heart: Always brush in the direction of your heart to promote lymphatic drainage. This means starting at your feet and brushing upwards towards your thighs.

3. Use Long Strokes on Limbs: For your legs and arms, use long, sweeping strokes. This technique helps improve circulation and encourages the movement of lymph fluids.
4. Circular Motions on the Torso: When you reach your abdomen, chest, and joints, use circular motions. This method is particularly effective for these areas as it stimulates deeper layers of skin and underlying tissues.
5. Be Gentle with Sensitive Areas: Apply less pressure on sensitive areas like your neck, breasts, and any areas where your skin feels delicate. The goal is to stimulate, not irritate.

Post-Brushing Care

1. Shower: After completing your dry brushing session, take a warm shower to rinse away the loosened skin cells and any toxins brought to the surface.
2. Moisturise: Post-shower, apply a nourishing moisturiser or body oil to hydrate your skin. This step is crucial as dry brushing can temporarily dry out your skin.
3. Hydrate Internally: Drink plenty of water to help flush out toxins and support overall skin health.

1. Agnivesha. In: Charaka, Dridhabala, Charaka Samhita, Sutra Sthana, 26/81. Reprint. Vaidya Jadavaji Trikamaji Acharya., editor. Varanasi: Krishnadas Academy; 2000. p. 149. [Google Scholar]

2. Ibid. Charaka Samhita, Sutra Sthana, 26/84. :150. [Google Scholar]

3. Ibid. Charaka Samhita, Sutra Sthana., 26/103. :151. [Google Scholar]

- "The 4. Complete Book of Ayurvedic Home Remedies" by Vasant Lad and "Ayurveda and the Mind" by David Frawley
- These texts explain the principles of Ayurveda, including the concept of doshas and the importance of maintaining skin health. Use them to understand the Ayurvedic perspective on skin care and how it relates to overall health and longevity.

A study by Granstein, Richard Detal, in the journal Neuroimmunology of the Skin, highlights that daily oil application on the skin maintains a healthy skin microbiome. This practice enhances our immune system by fostering communication between skin microbes, environmental microbes, and gut microbes, thereby supporting overall bodily functions. When the skin becomes dry, a common symptom of Vata dosha imbalance, the skin microbiome weakens, leading to diminished immunity, reduced longevity, and vitality. Therefore, safeguarding the skin, our body's largest organ inhabited by billions of microbes, emerges as a critical factor for health and longevity.

Chapter 7:
Let's Get Started: Your Yoga Journey Begins

Prepare your detox drink and drink it, as mentioned in previous chapter.

Day 1

You can sit with a straight spine, and a tall neck, and roll your shoulders back.

Sahaj Bhawasana

Neck rotation - 5 times clockwise and anti-clockwise

Shoulder rotation - 5 times Clockwise and 5 times anti-clockwise

Wrist rotation - 5 times clockwise and 5 times anti-clockwise

Waist rotation - Stand and rotate your waist 5 times clockwise and 5 times anti-clockwise

Ankle rotation (each leg) - 5 times clockwise and 5 times anti-clockwise

Warm-up

10 jumping jacks

10 leg raise-ups

10 squats

10 cross-body toe touch

10 mountain climbings

30 seconds plank hold

Asanas

Vrikshasana - (20 sec hold) on each leg.

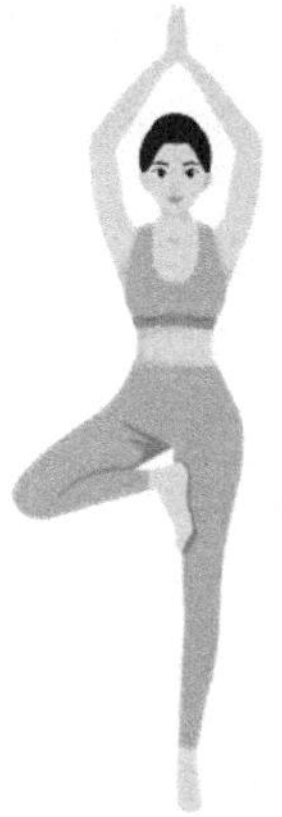

Veerbhadrasana 2 - (20 sec hold each side) on each side.

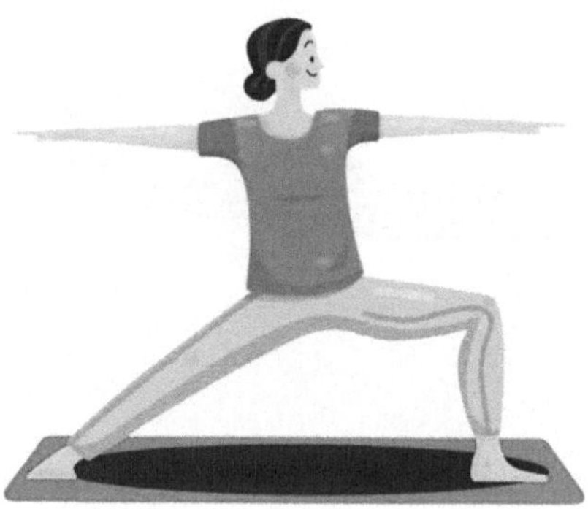

Parsvakonasana - (20 sec hold) on each side

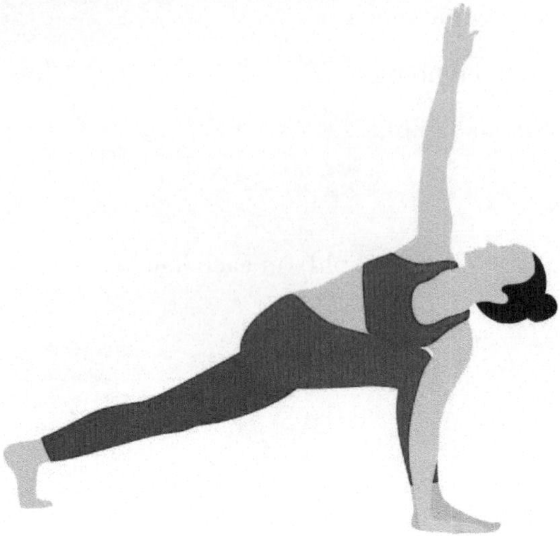

Bhujangasana - (20 sec hold)

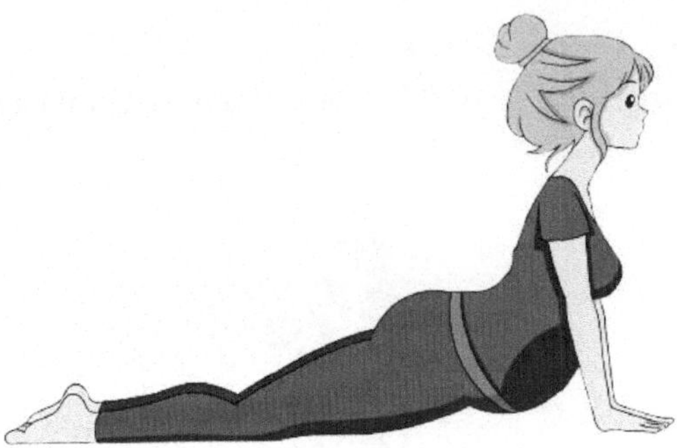

Balasana - (20 sec hold)

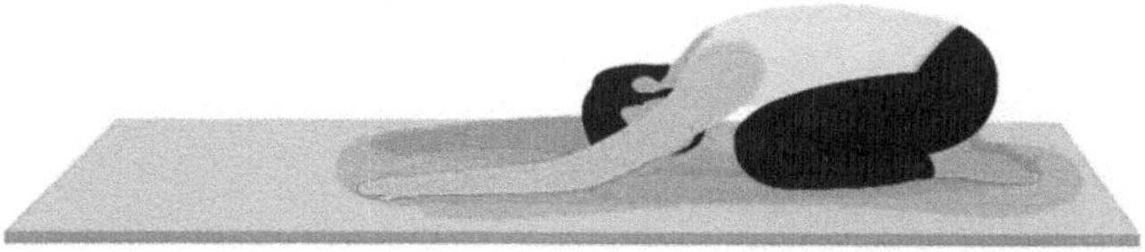

Vyaghrasana - (20 sec hold) on each side

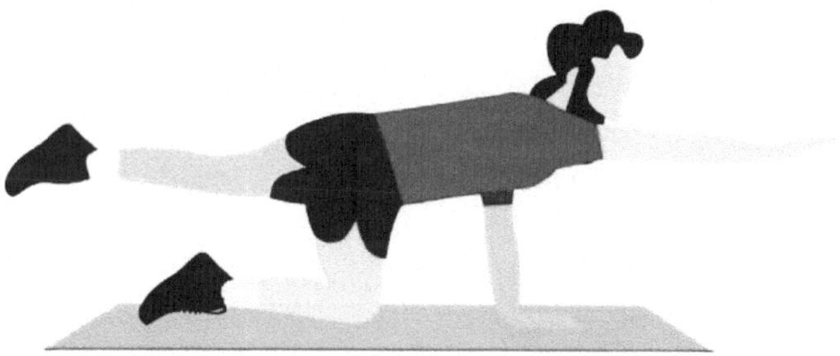

Bhaddakonasana- (Flapping for 30 sec)

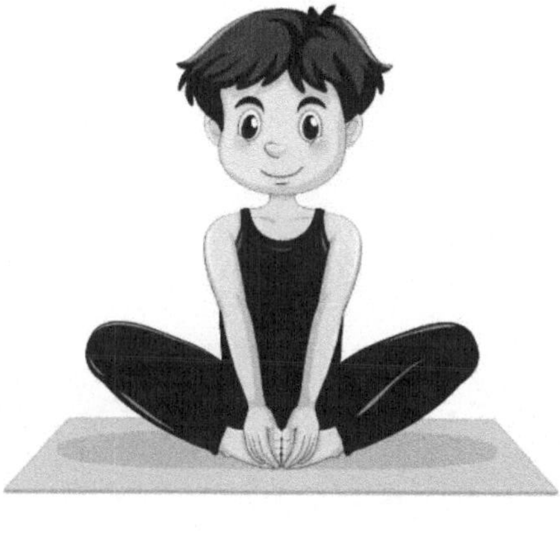

Anjaneyasana - (20 sec hold) on each side

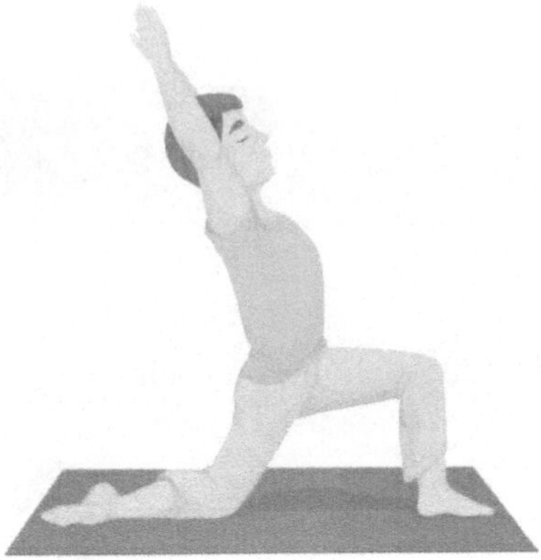

Dhanurasana - (20 sec hold)

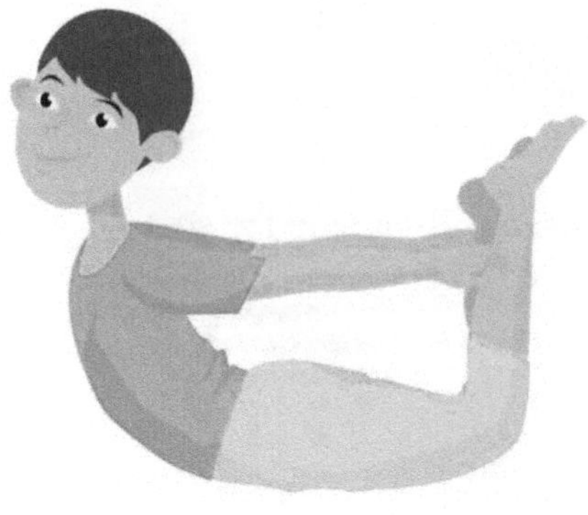

Savasana - 1 minute

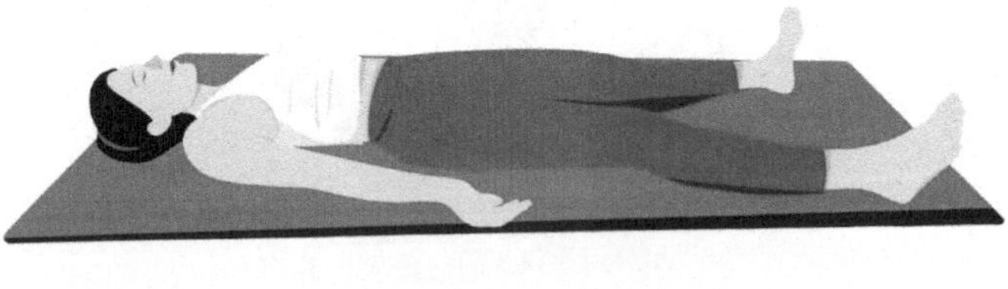

Sit for Pranayama

8 minutes Anulom vilom

- Sit in a relaxed posture with your spine straight.
- Close your eyes and rest your left hand on your knee.
- Use your right thumb to close your right nostril.
- Use your ring finger to close your left nostril when needed.

Breathing Pattern

- **Inhale deeply through the left nostril** while keeping the right nostril closed.
- **Close the left nostril** and open the right nostril, then **exhale completely** through the right nostril.
- **Inhale through the right nostril**, keeping the left nostril closed.
- **Close the right nostril** and open the left nostril, then **exhale through the left nostril**.

5 minutes Bhramari pranayama

- Sit in a quiet place with your spine straight.
- Close your eyes and take a few deep breaths to relax.
- Place your index fingers on your forehead.
- Use your middle and ring fingers to gently close your eyes.
- Place your thumbs over your ears to block external sounds.

Inhale Deeply Through the Nose

- Fill your lungs completely with air.
- As you exhale, make a deep humming sound like a bee ("mmm...").
- Feel the vibrations in your head and chest.

Meditation

Guided Savasana Body Scan Relaxation

1. Lie Down Comfortably
    - Lie flat on your back in Savasana (Corpse Pose).
    - Keep your arms relaxed by your sides, palms facing up.
    - Let your legs fall naturally apart.
2. Relax Your Body
    - Let go of any tension and allow your body to feel completely at ease.
    - Close your eyes and take slow, deep breaths.
3. Scan Your Body from Head to Toe
    - Bring your awareness to the top of your head. Observe any sensations for 2-5 seconds.
    - Move your attention slowly to your forehead, eyes, cheeks, and jaw, noticing any tightness.
    - Continue scanning down to your neck, shoulders, arms, hands, and fingers, allowing them to relax.
    - Shift focus to your chest, abdomen, and back, releasing any tension.
    - Move your awareness to your hips, thighs, knees, lower legs, ankles, and feet, feeling them completely at rest.

4. Stay in the Moment
    - Remain in this deeply relaxed state for 10 minutes.
    - Observe your breath and let go of any thoughts.
5. Gently Return
    - When ready, take a deep breath and slowly bring awareness back to your surroundings.
    - Move your fingers and toes, stretch gently, and open your eyes.

This practice helps calm the mind, relieve stress, and promote deep relaxation.

Day 2

Start your day with detox drink.

You can sit with straight spine, tall neck, roll your shoulders back.

Neck Exercise - Up and down - Left and Right - Bend side to side (5 times each)

Shoulder Exercise - Open your arms and fold them and start rotating clockwise and Anti - clockwise.

Wrist rotation - Stand and rotate your waist 5 times clockwise and 5 times anti - clockwise

Waist Rotation -Waist rotation - 5 times clockwise and 5 times anti - clockwise

Ankle rotation (each leg) - 5 times clockwise and 5 times anti -clockwise

Warm up

20 counts Ridha Gati(jogging)

10 leg raise up

10 squats

10 cross body toe touch

20 mountain climbings

1 minutes plank hold

Asanas

uttkatasana

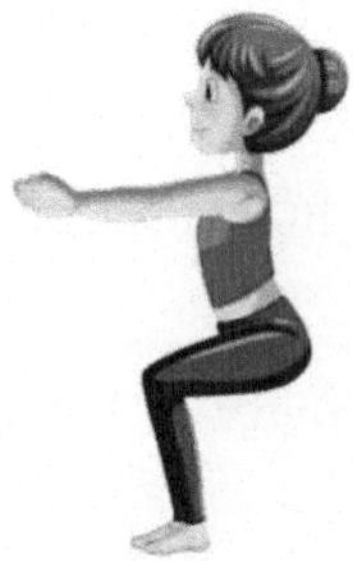

Veerbhadrasana 3 - (20 sec hold each side)

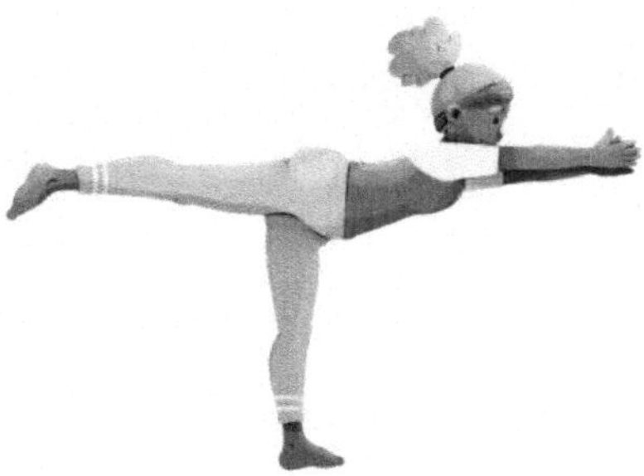

Navkasana - (30 sec hold each side)

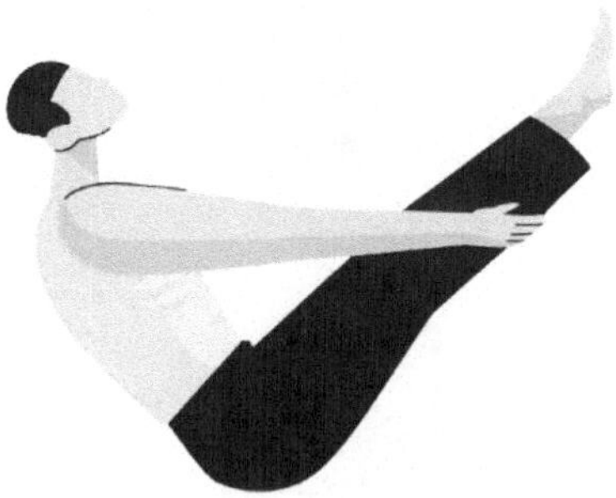

Bhaddakonasana- (Flapping for 30 sec)

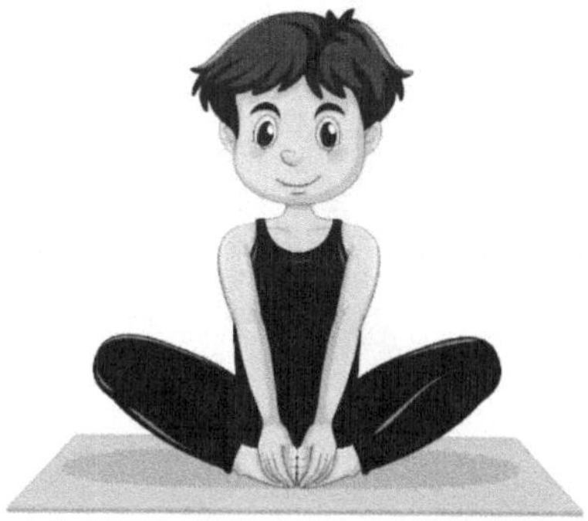

Setu Bandhasana- (30 sec hold)

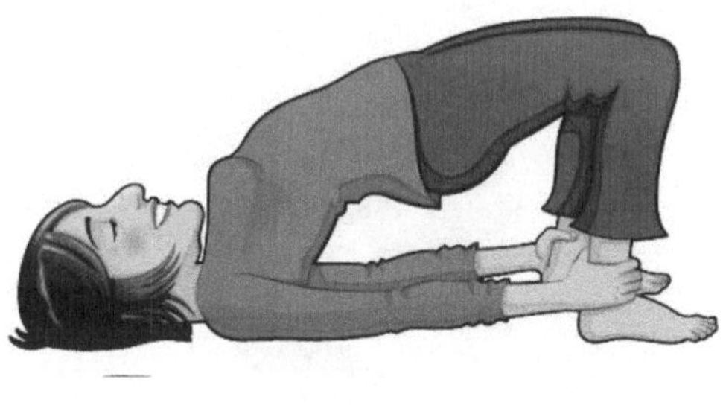

Ardha Matsyendrasana- (30 sec hold) on each side

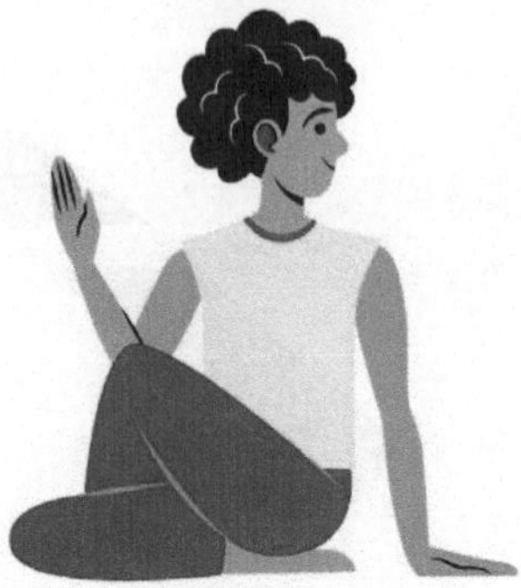

Sarvangasana - (20 sec hold)

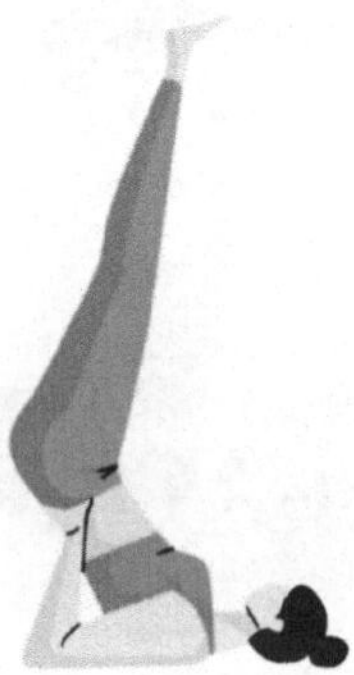

Halasana- (20 sec hold)

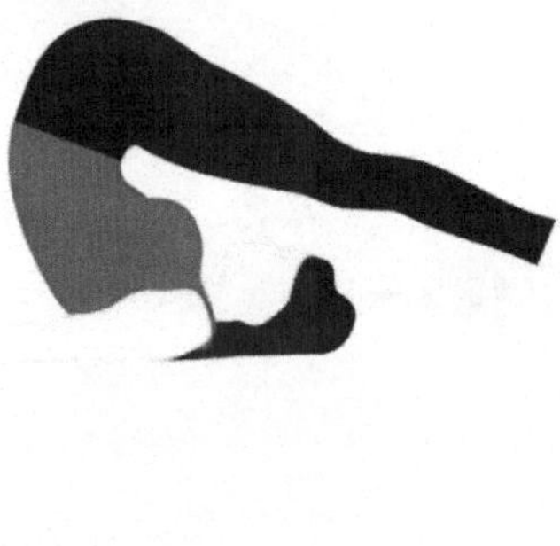

Malasana

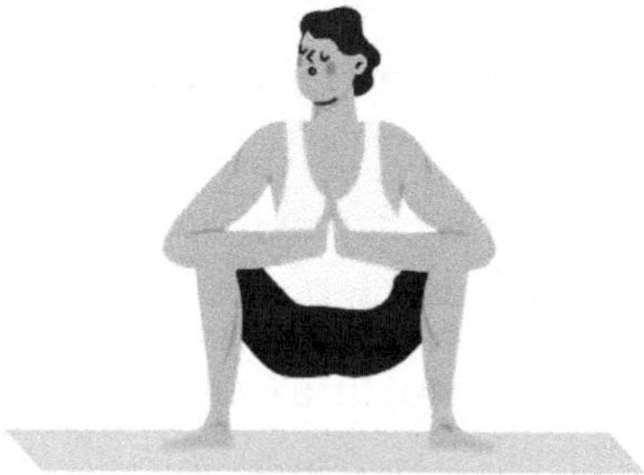

Savasana - 1 minute

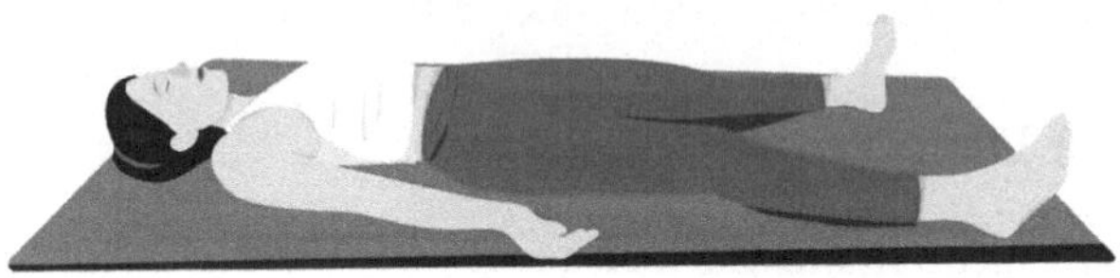

Sit for Pranayama

8 minutes Anulom vilom

- Sit in a relaxed posture with your spine straight.
- Close your eyes and rest your left hand on your knee.
- Use your right thumb to close your right nostril.
- Use your ring finger to close your left nostril when needed.

Breathing Pattern

- **Inhale deeply through the left nostril** while keeping the right nostril closed.

- **Close the left nostril** and open the right nostril, then **exhale completely** through the right nostril.
- **Inhale through the right nostril**, keeping the left nostril closed.
- **Close the right nostril** and open the left nostril, then **exhale through the left nostril**.

5 minutes udgeeth pranayama

- Sit comfortably in a cross-legged position with your spine straight.
- Close your eyes and relax your body.

Take a Deep Inhalation

- Breathe in slowly and deeply through your nose, filling your lungs completely.
- As you exhale, **chant "Aum" in a long, continuous tone**:
    - The **"A"** sound should be prolonged and deep.
    - The **"U"** sound should be vibrant enough to create vibration in your body.
    - Than “M” Sound should be soft and gentle.
- The exhalation should be **longer than the inhalation**.

Meditation

Find a quite and comfortable place to sit in sukhasana for meditation. Keep your hands in gyan mudra.

Start with taking really slow inhalations and then really slow exhalations.This brings the body in a calm & relaxed state really quickly. Now bring your full attention to the tip of your nose. Focus on the pattern of your breath. Feel the sensations of the air coming in & going out of your nostrils. Do not think about anything else right now. Be in this moment for 10 to 12 minutes on day

Day 3

Start your day with detox drink.

You can sit with straight spine, tall neck, roll your shoulders back.

Neck Exercise - Up and down - Left and Right - Bend side to side (5 times each)

Shoulder Exercise - Open your arms and fold them and start rotating clockwise and Anti - clockwise.

Wrist rotation - Stand and rotate your waist 5 times clockwise and 5 times anti - clockwise

Waist Rotation -Waist rotation - 5 times clockwise and 5 times anti - clockwise

Ankle rotation (each leg) - 5 times clockwise and 5 times anti -clockwise

Warm up

10 counts jumping jacks

10 high knee jumps

10 squats

10 cross body toe touch

20 mountain climbings

1 minutes plank hold

Asanas

uttkatasana

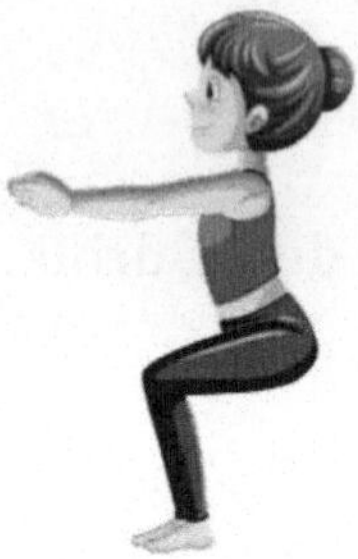

Veerbhadrasana 3 - (20 sec hold each side)

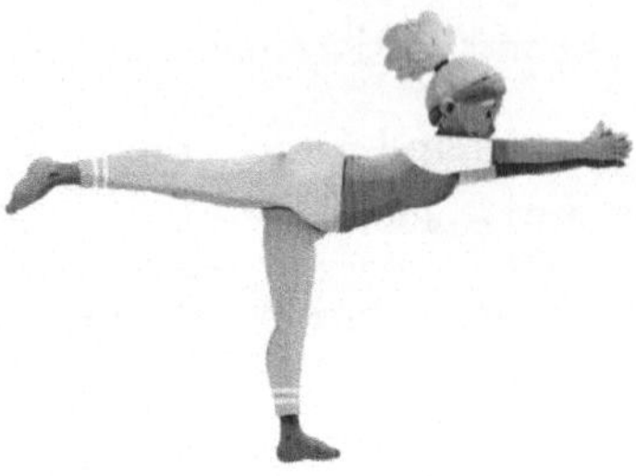

Navkasana - (30 sec hold each side)

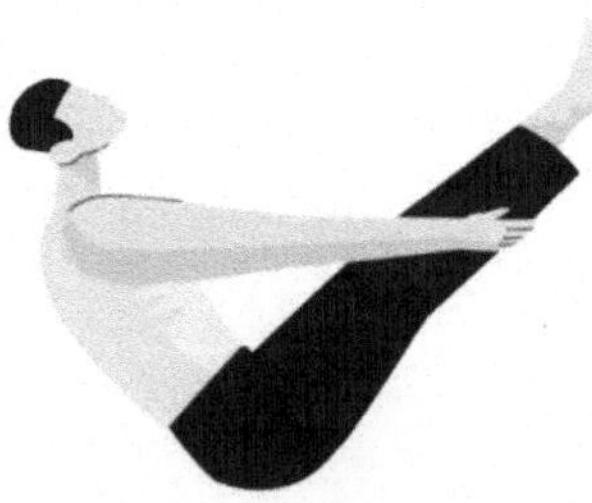

Bhaddakonasana- (Flapping for 30 sec)

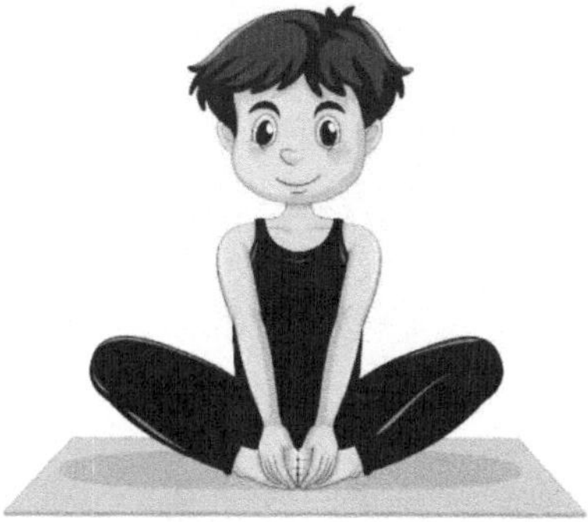

Setu Bandhasana- (30 sec hold)

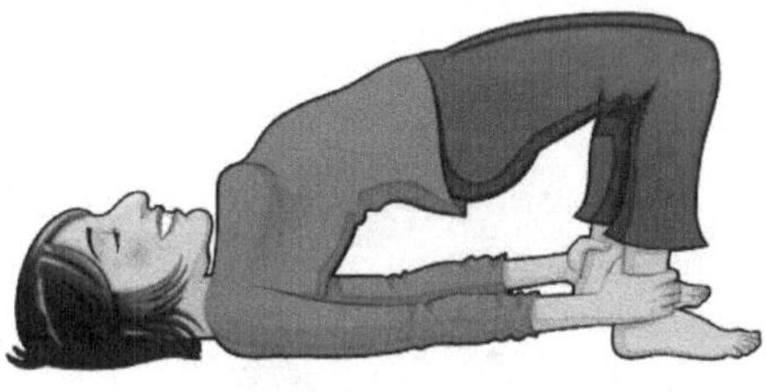

Ardha Matsyendrasana- (30 sec hold) on each side

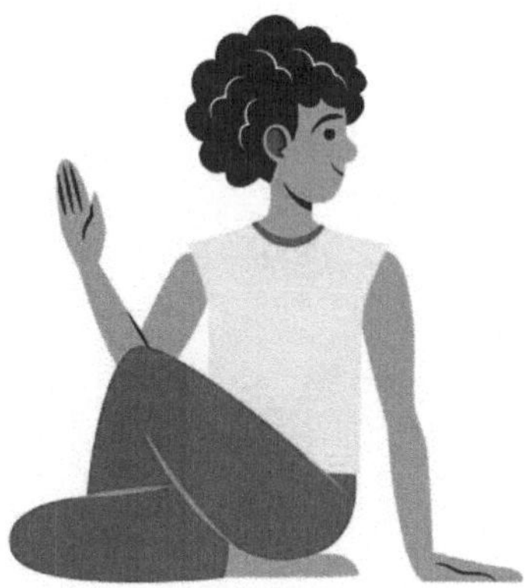

Sarvangasana - (20 sec hold)

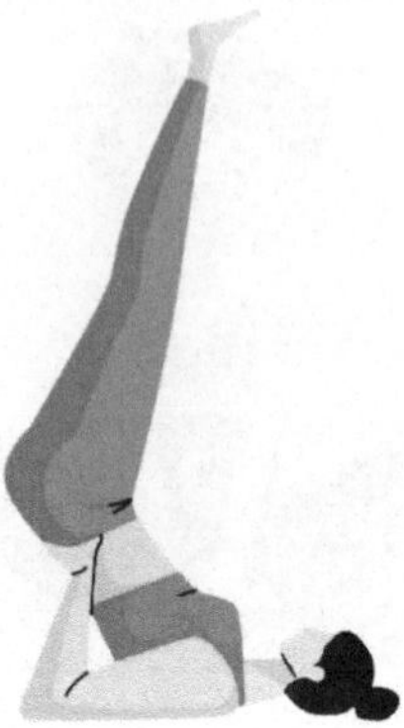

Halasana- (20 sec hold)

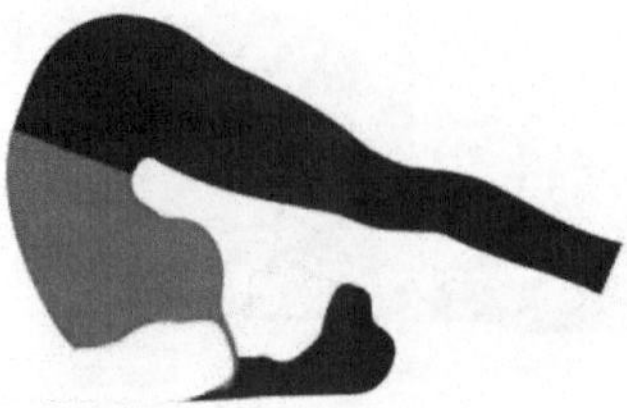

Malasana

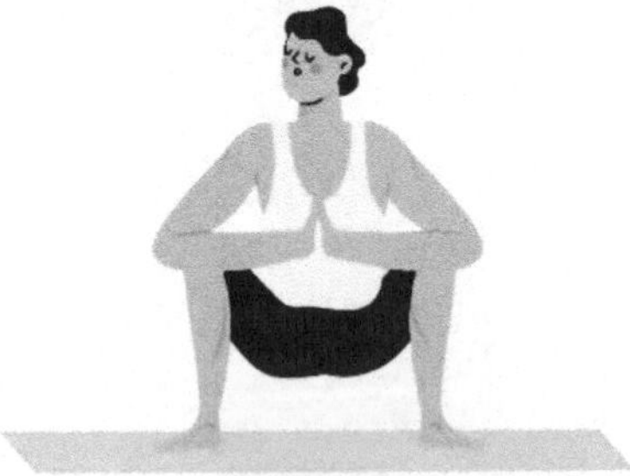

Savasana - 1 minute

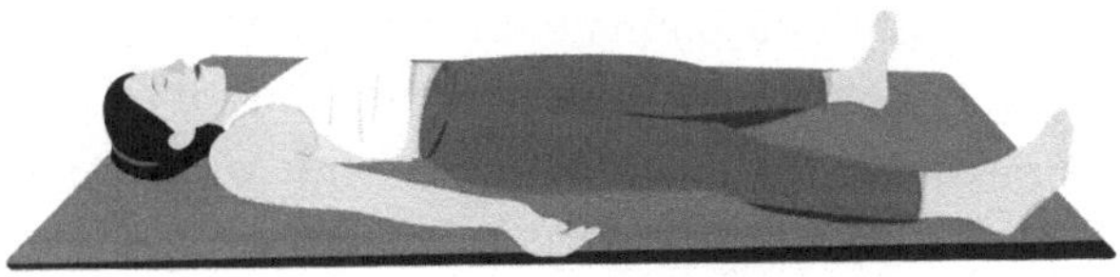

Sit for Pranayama

5 minutes samavriti (Box breathing)

- Sit in a relaxed posture with your spine straight.
- Close your eyes and take a few natural breaths to settle in.

Establish an Equal Breathing Pattern

- Inhale slowly through the nose for a count of **4**.
- Hold the breath for a count of **4**.
- Exhale smoothly through the nose for a count of **4**.
- Hold the breath again for a count of **4** before repeating the cycle.

Maintain a Rhythmic Flow

- Continue this pattern for **5 minutes**.
- If comfortable, gradually increase the count to **6 or 8** for deeper relaxation.

5 minutes Ujjai pranayama

- Sit in a relaxed yet upright posture with your spine straight.
- Close your eyes and take a few normal breaths to settle.

Constrict Your Throat Slightly

- Take a slow, deep inhale through your nose.
- As you inhale, gently contract the throat muscles (similar to fogging up a mirror with your breath, but with your mouth closed).
- This creates a soothing, ocean-like sound.

Slow & Controlled Exhalation

- Exhale slowly through the nose while maintaining the same throat constriction.
- Keep your breath steady and even, ensuring the same length for inhalation and exhalation.

Maintain a Rhythmic Flow

- Continue for 5 minutes, focusing on the sound and sensation of your breath.

Meditation

Find a quiet and comfortable place to sit in sukhasana for meditation. Keep your hands one on the other

Start with taking slow inhalations and then really slow exhalations. This brings the body to a calm & relaxed state quickly. Now bring your full attention to the tip of your nose. Focus on the pattern of your breath. Feel the sensations of the air coming in & going out of your nostrils. Do not think about anything else right now. Be in this moment for 10 to 12 minutes on the day

Day 4

Start your day with detox drink.

You can sit with a straight spine, and tall neck, and roll your shoulders back.

Neck Exercise - Up and down - Left and Right - Bend side to side (5 times each)

Shoulder Exercise - Open your arms fold them and start rotating clockwise and Anti-clockwise.

Wrist rotation - 5 times clockwise and 5 times anti-clockwise

Waist Rotation -Waist rotation - 5 times clockwise and 5 times anti-clockwise

Ankle rotation (each leg) - 5 times clockwise and 5 times anti-clockwise

Warm-up

Warm-up

10 jumping jacks

10 leg raise-ups

10 squats

10 cross-body toe touch

10 mountain climbings

1 minutes plank hold

Asanas

Natrajasana - (20 sec hold each leg)

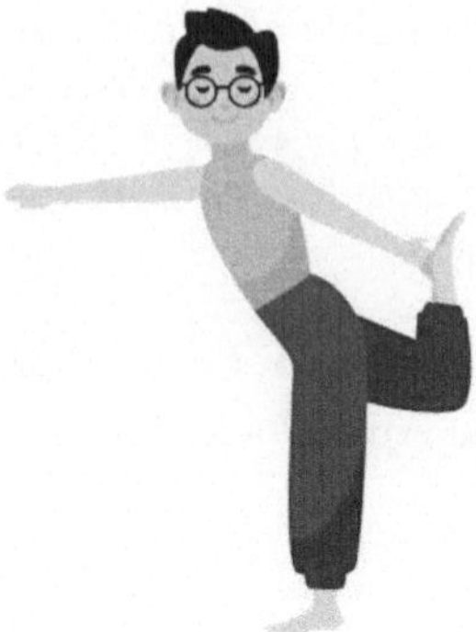

Veerbhadrasana 3 - (20 sec hold each side)

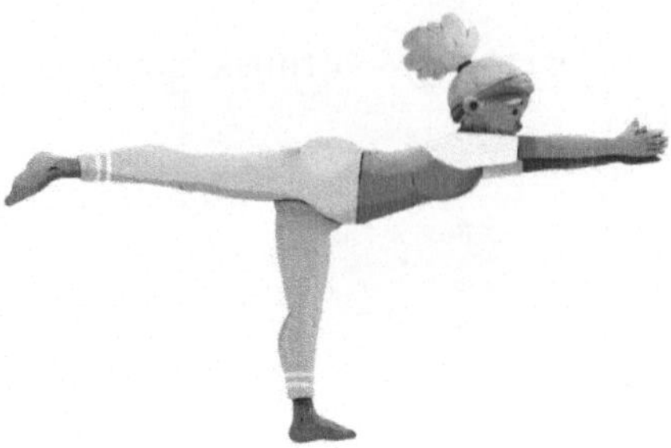

Kumbhakasana

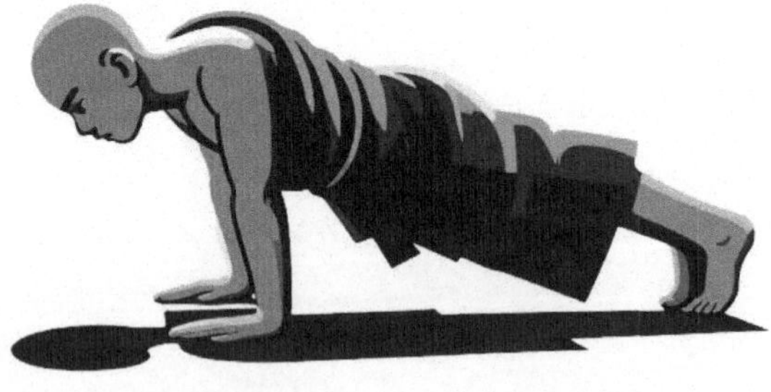

Ustrasana

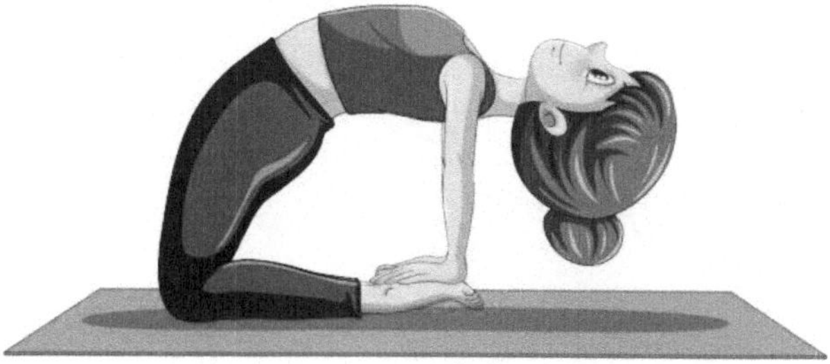

Parsva upavistha konasana - (20 sec hold)

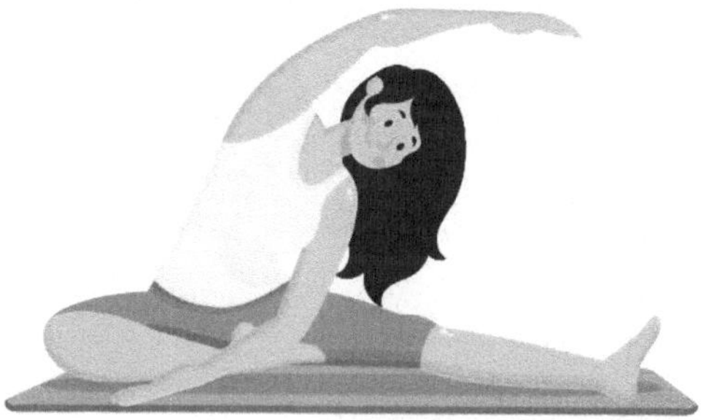

Halasana- (20 sec hold)

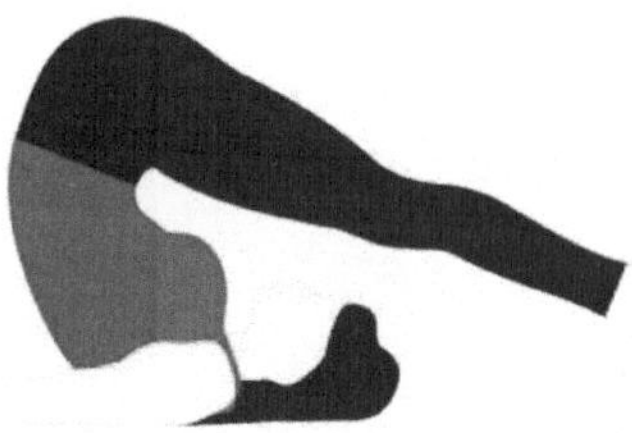

Dhanurasana - (20 sec hold)

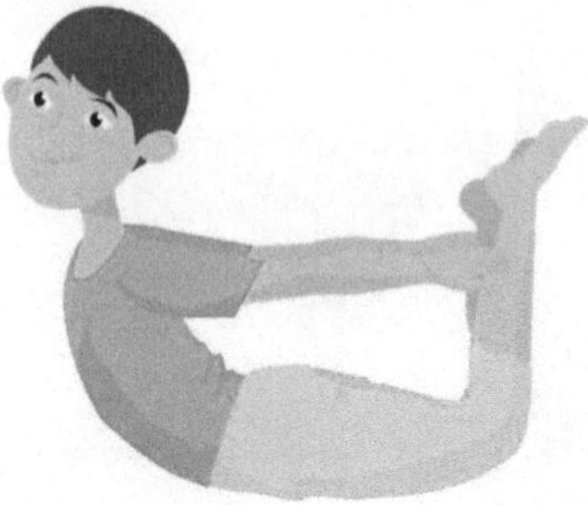

Savasana - 1 minute

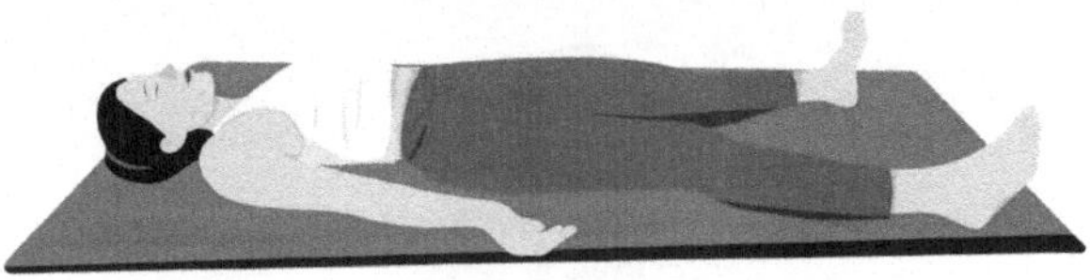

Sit for Pranayama

5 minutes Anulom vilom

- Sit in a relaxed posture with your spine straight.
- Close your eyes and rest your left hand on your knee.
- Use your right thumb to close your right nostril.
- Use your ring finger to close your left nostril when needed.

Breathing Pattern

- **Inhale deeply through the left nostril** while keeping the right nostril closed.
- **Close the left nostril** and open the right nostril, then **exhale completely** through the right nostril.

- **Inhale through the right nostril**, keeping the left nostril closed.
- **Close the right nostril** and open the left nostril, then **exhale through the left nostril**.
- Continue this cycle for 5 minutes, focusing on slow, deep breaths.
-

3 minutes Ujjai pranayama

- Sit in a relaxed yet upright posture with your spine straight.
- Close your eyes and take a few normal breaths to settle.

Constrict Your Throat Slightly

- Take a slow, deep inhale through your nose.
- As you inhale, gently contract the throat muscles (similar to fogging up a mirror with your breath, but with your mouth closed).
- This creates a soothing, ocean-like sound.
- Exhale slowly through the nose while maintaining the same throat constriction.
- Keep your breath steady and even, ensuring the same length for inhalation and exhalation.
- Continue for 5 minutes, focusing on the sound and sensation of your breath.

Meditation

Find a quite and comfortable place to sit in sukhasana for meditation. Keep your hands one on other

Start with taking really slow inhalations and then really slow exhalations. This brings the body in a calm & relaxed state really quickly. Now bring your full attention to the tip of your nose. Focus on the pattern of your breath. Feel the sensations of the air coming in & going out of your nostrils. Do not think about anything else right now. Be in this moment for 10 to 12 minutes.

Day 5

Start your day with detox drink.

You can sit with a straight spine, and tall neck, and roll your shoulders back.

Neck Exercise - Up and down - Left and Right - Bend side to side (5 times each)

Shoulder Exercise - Open your arms fold them and start rotating clockwise and Anti-clockwise.

Wrist rotation - 5 times clockwise and 5 times anti-clockwise

Waist Rotation -Waist rotation - 5 times clockwise and 5 times anti-clockwise

Ankle rotation (each leg) - 5 times clockwise and 5 times anti-clockwise

Warm-up

10 counts jumping jacks

10 high knee jumps

10 squats

10 cross body toe touch

20 mountain climbings

1 minutes plank hold

Asanas

Devisana

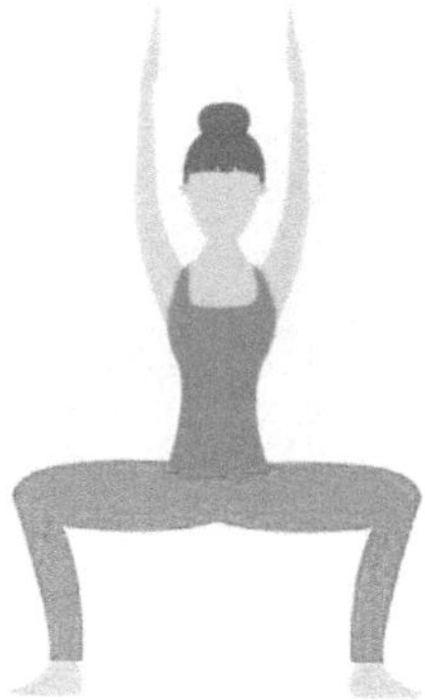

Paschimottanasana

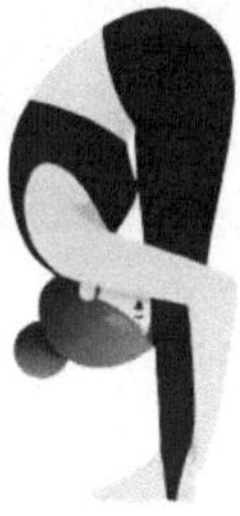

Trikonasana - (20 sec hold each side)

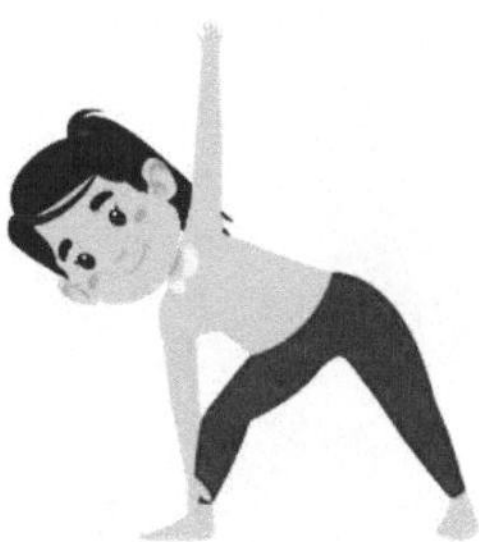

Gomukhasana

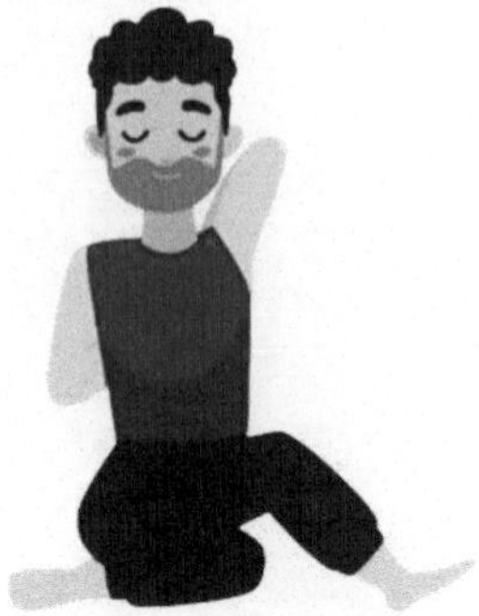

Kumbhakasana

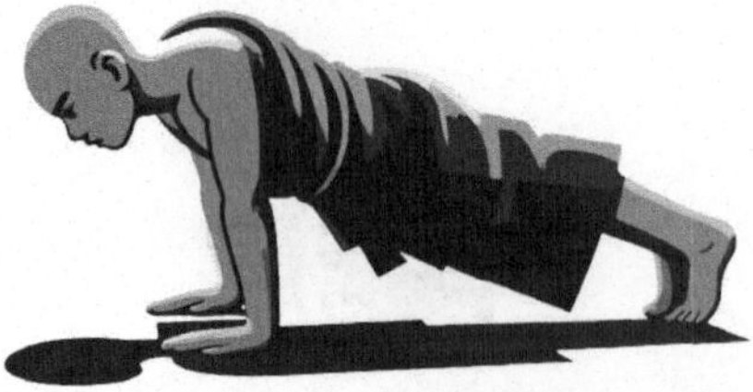

Sarvangasana - (20 sec hold)

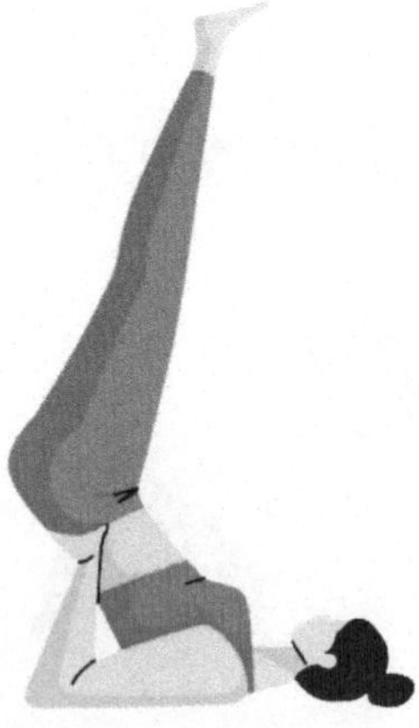

Dhanurasana - (20 sec hold)

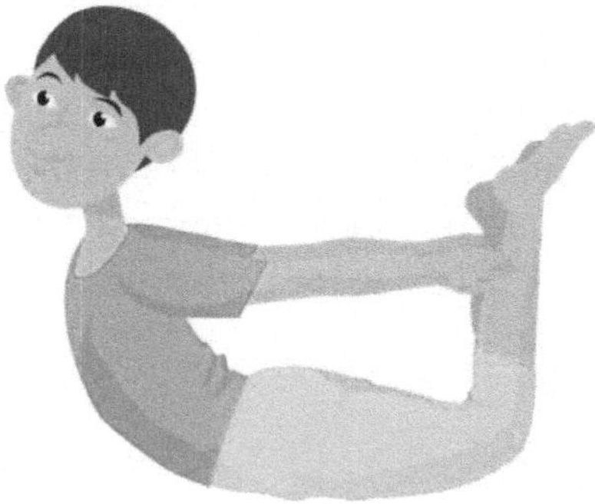

Savasana - 1 minute

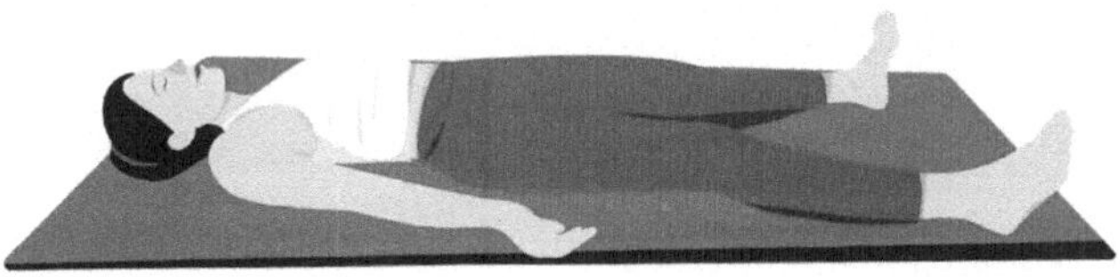

Sit for Pranayama

5 minutes Anulom vilom

- Sit in a relaxed posture with your spine straight.
- Close your eyes and rest your left hand on your knee.
- Use your right thumb to close your right nostril.
- Use your ring finger to close your left nostril when needed.

Breathing Pattern

- **Inhale deeply through the left nostril** while keeping the right nostril closed.

- **Close the left nostril** and open the right nostril, then **exhale completely** through the right nostril.
- **Inhale through the right nostril**, keeping the left nostril closed.
- **Close the right nostril** and open the left nostril, then **exhale through the left nostril**.
- Continue this cycle for 5 minutes, focusing on slow, deep breaths.

5 minutes samavriti (Box breathing)

- Sit in a relaxed posture with your spine straight.
- Close your eyes and take a few natural breaths to settle in.

Establish an Equal Breathing Pattern

- Inhale slowly through the nose for a count of **4**.
- Hold the breath for a count of **4**.
- Exhale smoothly through the nose for a count of **4**.
- Hold the breath again for a count of **4** before repeating the cycle.

Maintain a Rhythmic Flow

- Continue this pattern for **5 minutes**.
- If comfortable, gradually increase the count to **6 or 8** for deeper relaxation.